Veterinary Medical School Admission Requirements

Veterinary Medical School Admission Requirements

2017 EDITION FOR 2018 MATRICULATION

ASSOCIATION OF AMERICAN VETERINARY MEDICAL COLLEGES

PURDUE UNIVERSITY PRESS | WEST LAFAYETTE, INDIANA

Please be aware that the admission requirements described in this book are subject to change by individual institutions without prior notice. Additionally, while VMCAS has made every effort to ensure the accuracy of the information contained in this book, VMCAS is not liable for any misrepresentations of a college's requirements. The provisions of this book do not constitute a contract between any applicant or student and the colleges of veterinary medicine.

Compiled by the Association of American Veterinary Medical Colleges;
Tony Wynne, Editor, Director of Admissions and Recruitment Affairs

Cover photograph courtesy of Virginia-Maryland College of Veterinary Medicine.
Back cover photographs courtesy of Lincoln Memorial University and Mississippi State University.

Paperback ISBN: 978-1-55753-786-7
ePub ISBN: 978-1-61249-505-7
ePDF ISBN: 978-1-61249-504-0
ISSN: 1089-6465

ACCEPTANCE DATE POLICY

In order to grant member schools enough time to complete their admissions processes and to give applicants enough time to consider all offers of admissions, no AAVMC Member Institution will require any applicant to make a decision about admission or financial aid before April 15 of each year. If April 15 falls on a Saturday or a Sunday, the date will be shifted to the following Monday.

To ensure applicants are awareness of this policy, each Member Institution will attach a copy of this policy to all admissions offer letters.

This policy does not apply to:
- Institutions outside the U.S. that do not participate in VMCAS
- Offers of admission for non-VMCAS applicants to institutions outside the U.S.
- Offers of admission for matriculation that is other than August or September

PROCEDURE

The Executive Director will investigate all complaints about alleged violations of this policy and report any findings to the chair of the Admissions and Recruitment Committee.

First Offense: If a Member Institution is found to be in violation of the policy, the Executive Director will send a Warning Letter to the Dean and Admissions Director of the institution and inform the Executive Committee of the Board of Directors.

Second and Subsequent Offenses: If a Member Institution is found to be in violation of this policy after a Warning Letter has been issued, the Executive Director and the chair of the Admissions and Recruitment Committee will report their findings to the Board of Directors and make a recommendation for additional penalties. Penalties may include monetary fines and exclusion from participation in VMCAS for a specified period of time.

Approved by the AAVMC Board of Directors
November 10, 2014

CONTENTS

FOREWORD

Congratulations on your decision to prepare for a career in veterinary medicine. Veterinary medicine is an exciting and rewarding career that provides a diverse array of options for contributing to the health of animals, people, and the planet.

Published annually by the Association of American Veterinary Medical Colleges (AAVMC), this *Veterinary Medical School Admission Requirements (VMSAR)* publication helps prospective students consider an important mix of factors when preparing for a veterinary medical education, including cost, financial aid, special programs, standardized tests, the AAVMC Veterinary Medical College Application Service (VMCAS), and the various colleges and schools' residency admissions requirements.

Where to apply and attend will be one of your initial decisions, and it's an important one, but all of these American Veterinary Medical Association (AVMA)-accredited schools offer great programs. Each one can start you on a rewarding path filled with choices and opportunities. Animal clinical care is an important and popular option in veterinary medicine, but veterinarians also contribute to global health in many other ways, including through careers in public health, research, and specialty practice. You also can prepare yourself for scientific and administrative careers with pharmaceutical, nutrition, and biomedical health corporations, or work in state and federal government. Augmenting your professional degree with advanced graduate work can lead to faculty positions in higher education.

> Our profession offers many opportunities beyond the time-honored practice of providing clinical care in general practice.

Like other health professions, the pursuit and achievement of a veterinary medical education represents a substantial investment of time, effort, and financial resources. Cost-saving strategies include focusing on in-state veterinary medical schools or states that offer in-state tuition as part of special agreements with neighboring states. Other strategies include focusing on areas of greatest need, such as rural veterinary practice where loan repayment options might be available.

More information can be found on individual college and school websites or on the AAVMC website at www.aavmc.org. Prospective students also can contact the appropriate admissions office at each school or the VMCAS Student and Advisor Hotline, either by e-mail (vmcasinfo@vmcas.org) or by calling VMCAS at (617) 612-2884. The Veterinary Student Engagement System (VSES) is a useful tool as well.

Perhaps no other medical career provides such a broad base of biomedical training and leads to so many different areas of opportunity. The choices can seem overwhelming, but this guide is a great place to start, and step by step, your path will become clear, as it did for me. In my own case, a veterinary medical education led me to service as an officer in the United States Air Force, work in a mixed animal practice, in public health as an official with the U.S. Centers for Disease Control and Prevention, and now, as executive director of the AAVMC.

All of us at the AAVMC wish you luck and success as you prepare yourself for service in this extraordinary profession.

Dr. Andrew Maccabe
AAVMC Chief Executive Officer

ABOUT THE AAVMC

The Association of American Veterinary Medical Colleges (AAVMC) is a non-profit membership organization working to protect and improve the health and welfare of animals, people, and the environment by advancing academic veterinary medicine. The association was founded in 1966 by the deans of the then-existing eighteen colleges of veterinary medicine in the United States and three in Canada. During the 1970s and 1980s, AAVMC's membership expanded to include departments of veterinary science in colleges of agriculture, and in the 1990s to include divisions or departments of comparative medicine. In 2008, AAVMC began accepting non-accredited colleges and schools of veterinary medicine as affiliate members.

Today, AAVMC provides leadership for an academic veterinary medical community that includes all thirty colleges of veterinary medicine in the United States; nine departments of veterinary science; eight departments of comparative medicine; all five veterinary medical colleges in Canada; thirteen accredited colleges of veterinary medicine in Australia, Grenada, Ireland, Mexico, the Netherlands, New Zealand, St. Kitts, the United Kingdom, and six affiliate members.

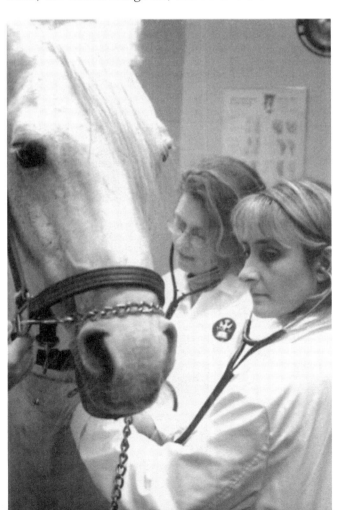

MISSION

AAVMC provides leadership for and promotes excellence in academic veterinary medicine to prepare the veterinary workforce with the scientific knowledge and skills required to meet societal needs through the protection of animal health, the relief of animal suffering, the conservation of animal resources, the promotion of public health, and the advancement of medical knowledge.

AAVMC pursues its mission by providing leadership in:
- Advocating on behalf of academic veterinary medicine;
- Serving as a catalyst and convener on issues of importance to academic veterinary medicine;
- Providing information, knowledge, and solutions to support members' work;
- Facilitating enrollment in veterinary medical schools and colleges; and
- Building global partnerships and coalitions to advance our collective goals.

STRATEGIC GOALS

1. Lead efforts to review, evaluate, and improve veterinary medical education in order to prepare graduates with the competencies needed to address societal needs.
2. Lead efforts to increase the amount of veterinary research conducted and the number of graduates entering research careers.
3. Lead efforts to recruit a student body aligned with the demands for veterinary expertise.
4. Lead efforts to increase the number of racially and/or ethnically underrepresented in veterinary medicine (URVM*) individuals throughout academic veterinary medicine.
5. Lead efforts to develop the next generation of leaders for academic veterinary medicine.
6. Strengthen AAVMC's capacity to better serve its members, partners, and other stakeholders in advancing the AAVMC mission.

*"URVMs are populations of individuals whose advancement in the veterinary medical profession have historically been disproportionately impacted by six specific aspects of diversity (gender, race, ethnicity, and geographic, socio-economic, and educational disadvantage) due to legal, cultural, or social climate impediments." *Definition of Underrepresented in Veterinary Medicine (URVM)*, approved by the AAVMC Board of Directors, July 20, 2008.

Left: A Tufts University Cummings School of Veterinary Medicine student checks out a horse with advice from her professor. Photo courtesy of Andy Cunningham of the Tufts University Cummings School of Veterinary Medicine.

VETERINARY MEDICINE: OPPORTUNITIES AND CHOICES

Veterinarians help animals and people live longer, healthier lives. They serve society through the protection of animal health and welfare, the prevention and relief of animal suffering, the conservation of animal resources, the promotion of public health, and the advancement of medical knowledge. The Doctor of Veterinary Medicine degree can lead to diverse career opportunities and different lifestyles from a solo mixed-animal practice in a rural area to a teaching or research position at an urban university, medical center, or industrial laboratory. The majority of veterinarians in the United States are in private clinical practice, although significant numbers are involved in preventive medicine, regulatory veterinary medicine, military veterinary medicine, laboratory animal medicine, research and development in industry, and teaching and research in a variety of basic science and clinical disciplines.

THE SPECTRUM OF OPPORTUNITIES IN VETERINARY MEDICINE

Veterinarians may choose to become specialists in a clinical area or to work with particular species. The first step on the path toward specialization is usually an internship.

1) FURTHER TRAINING

Internship

Internships are one-year programs in either small- or large-animal medicine and surgery. The most prestigious internship programs are at veterinary medical colleges or at very large private veterinary hospitals with board-certified veterinarians on staff. Since internships are usually at large referral centers, interns are exposed to a larger number of challenging cases than they would be likely to see in a smaller private practice.

Veterinary students in their senior year and veterinary graduates apply for internships through a matching program. Internship applicants and training hospitals rank each other in order of preference, and a computerized system matches each applicant with the highest-ranking teaching hospital that ranked the applicant. Academic performance in the veterinary professional curriculum, as well as recommendations from veterinary school faculty, is considered in the ranking of internship applicants.

Most veterinary interns in the United States receive a nominal salary, and their educational debts, if any, may be postponed in some governmentally subsidized loan programs. Veterinarians can sometimes command a higher starting salary in private practice after completion of an internship. Also, an internship is often the next step, after receiving the veterinary degree, toward residency and board certification.

Residency Training

Residency training is more specialized than an internship. Residency training programs are competitive and most require that the prospective residents complete an internship or equivalent private-practice experience prior to beginning the residency programs. Residency training is available in disciplines as varied as internal medicine, surgery, preventive medicine, behavior, toxicology, dentistry, and pathology.

The programs take two to three years to complete, depending on the nature of the specialty. Successful completion of a residency often is an important step toward attainment of board certification. Some residencies combine research and graduate study, leading to master's or PhD degrees.

Board Certification

Currently, there are twenty-two AVMA-recognized veterinary specialty organizations, comprising forty distinct specialties: anesthesiology, animal behavior, clinical pharmacology, dentistry, dermatology, emergency and critical care, internal medicine, laboratory animal medicine, microbiology, nutrition, ophthalmology, pathology, poultry medicine, private practice, preventive medicine, radiology, surgery, sports medicine and rehabilitation, theriogenology (reproduction), toxicology, and zoological medicine. Veterinarians may become board certified by completing rigorous postgraduate training, education, and examination requirements.

2) PRIVATE AND PUBLIC PRACTICE

The majority of veterinary graduates are engaged in private practice, either as an owner of a solo practice or, more likely, as a partner or associate in a group practice. Increasingly, veterinarians work together as a team, which allows a wider range of services to be provided.

Small-animal veterinarians focus their efforts primarily on dogs and cats but are seeing a growing number of other pets, including other small mammals, birds, reptiles, and fish.

Large-animal veterinarians often place their emphasis on horses, cattle, or pigs, and work both on a farm-call and an in-clinic basis. A mixed-animal veterinarian works with all types of domestic animals.

Public practice provides a variety of opportunities at the international, national, state, county, or city levels. There are exciting career opportunities for veterinarians in food safety, public health, the military, animal disease control, and research. Some veterinarians are employed by zoos and aquariums, wildlife conservation groups, game farms, or fisheries.

3) INDUSTRY

Veterinarians have many opportunities available to them in private industry, particularly in the fields of nutrition and pharmaceuticals. Assisting in the development of new products in the animal industry, conducting research for pharmaceutical companies, diagnosing disease and drug effects as pathologists, or safeguarding the health of laboratory animal colonies are all interesting career possibilities.

4) CONCLUSION

By the very nature of the comparative medical education that veterinarians receive, the many species of animals they care for and work for, and the wide variety of clientele served, the opportunities available to today's veterinarian are abundant.

INFORMATION ABOUT STANDARDIZED TESTS

Most veterinary medical colleges require one or more standardized tests: the Graduate Record Examination (GRE) or the Medical College Admission Test (MCAT). For further information regarding test dates and registration procedures, contact the testing agencies listed below:

GRE Graduate Record Examinations
P.O. Box 6000
Princeton, NJ 08541-6000
(609) 771-7670 (Princeton, NJ)
also: (510) 654-1200 (Oakland, CA)
www.gre.org
Individual school codes: see GRE booklet

MCAT Medical College Admission Test
MCAT Program Office
P.O. Box 4056
Iowa City, IA 52243-4056
(319) 337-1357
www.aamc.org/students/applying/mcat

TOEFL Test of English as a Foreign Language
TOEFL/TSE Services
P.O. Box 6151
Princeton, NJ 08541-6151
(609) 771-7100
www.toefl.org

AAVMC MEMBER INSTITUTIONS AND THE ROLE OF ACCREDITATION

Veterinary Schools join the AAVMC as institutional or affiliate members. A key difference between these two membership categories is whether a college/school of veterinary medicine is accredited by the American Veterinary Medical Association's Council on Education (AVMA/COE). Only AVMA/COE-accredited colleges of veterinary medicine may join AAVMC as an institutional (voting) member. Colleges of veterinary medicine that are not AVMA-accredited may join AAVMC as an affiliate member (non-voting) only. Several of AAVMC's affiliate members (non-AVMA/COE-accredited institutions) have entered into agreements with AAVMC institutional members for clinical training. It is important for prospective veterinary students to know the different implications of attending and/or graduating from AVMA/COE-accredited vs. non-AVMA/COE-accredited colleges of veterinary medicine as it pertains to educational options and eventually seeking and obtaining a license to practice veterinary medicine. AAVMC encourages its affiliate members to become AVMA/COE-accredited.

ACCREDITATION

The AVMA/COE accredits DVM or equivalent educational programs. Accreditation through the AVMA/COE assures that minimum standards in veterinary medical education are met by accredited colleges of veterinary medicine and that students enrolled in these colleges receive an education that will prepare them for entry-level positions in the profession. In the United States, graduation from an AVMA/COE-accredited college of veterinary medicine is an important prerequisite for application for licensure. Internationally, some veterinary schools have chosen to seek AVMA/COE accreditation in addition to accreditation by the competent authority in their own regions. AVMA/COE accreditation of international veterinary schools provides assurance that those programs of education meet the same standards as other similarly accredited schools.

Additionally, AVMA/COE accreditation assures:

- Prospective students that they will meet a competency threshold for entry into practice, including eligibility for professional credentialing and/or licensure;
- Employers that graduates have achieved specified learning goals and are prepared to begin professional practice;
- Faculty, deans, and administrators that their programs measure satisfactorily against national standards and their own stated missions and goals;
- The public that public health and safety concerns are being addressed; and
- The veterinary profession that the science and art of veterinary medicine are being advanced through contemporary curricula.

*Source: The source for this information and a site recommended for obtaining additional information is as follows: https://www.avma.org/ProfessionalDevelopment/Education/Accreditation/Colleges/Pages/about-accred.aspx

LICENSURE

Licensure in the United States

In the United States, requirements for licensure are set by individual state regulatory boards. The North American Veterinary Licensing Exam (NAVLE) and any additional state exams must be taken by a graduate to become eligible for state licensure. The NAVLE, which is administered by the National Board of Veterinary Medical Examiners (NBVME), fulfills a core requirement for licensure to practice veterinary medicine in all jurisdictions in the United States and Canada. Mexico does not require NAVLE. In addition to the NAVLE, state regulatory boards will have other licensure requirements, which may include state-specific examinations.

To be eligible to take the NAVLE, applicants must have graduated from either an AVMA/COE-accredited college of veterinary medicine or a non-AVMA/COE-accredited college (see following details).

Applicants who graduated from a non-AVME/COE-accredited college must also have a certification of eligibility, which can come from one of two sources: the Educational Commission for Foreign Veterinary Graduates (ECFVG) Certification Program (www.avma.org/professionaldevelopment/education/foreign/pages/default.aspx) or the Program for the Assessment of Veterinary Education Equivalence (PAVE) (www.aavsb.org/PAVE).

All state regulatory boards accept the ECFVG certification, administered through the AVMA, as meeting in full or in part the educational prerequisite for licensure eligibility. At this time, twenty-eight state regulatory boards also accept PAVE certification, which is administered through the American Association of Veterinary State Boards (AAVSB).

It is important to note that prerequisites for licensure eligibility and requirements for licensure vary amongst state regulatory boards and are subject to periodic modification.

Licensure Outside the United States

Mutual recognition arrangements apply to jurisdictions where there are AVMA/COE-accredited schools. These specify that graduates of AVMA/COE-accredited schools in the United States and Canada are permitted to obtain licensure to practice under terms no less favorable than graduates of schools accredited by the competent authority in that jurisdiction.

DECIDING WHERE TO APPLY

There are several factors, as well as the issue of accreditation, that an applicant must consider in identifying school(s) to submit an application for admissions. In addition to licensure issues, there may be economic, educational options, or other differences that students should consider in making decisions on where to apply. This book is intended to provide important information about AAVMC members to assist in informed decision-making for students considering applying to one or more veterinary colleges.

VETERINARIAN PROFILE: LAURA NELSON

YEAR OF GRADUATION
2003

PLACE OF EMPLOYMENT
Michigan State University College of Veterinary Medicine

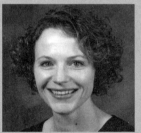

What is your favorite aspect of being a veterinarian?
In my role as a small animal surgeon, I love working with a team of experts to provide the best comprehensive care for my patients and their families. There is much more to surgery than surgery, and having excellent colleagues makes me more effective in my practice. As a veterinary educator, helping veterinary students develop the skills and practices needed to start their surgical careers is a joy and a tremendous privilege. I have the lucky job of training the future of the profession.

What type of veterinary medicine do you practice?
I am an academic small animal general surgeon.

Where did you attend veterinary school?
The Ohio State University.

How long have you been practicing as a veterinarian?
Almost 13 years! It goes fast.

What advice do you have for those considering a career in veterinary medicine?
It can be a challenging job, which is mostly a good thing. I would advise those considering it as a career to keep an open mind about the many possibilities within the profession. There are lots of ways to be a veterinarian and all are important. Let your goals change as you find out what you love. Finally, be mindful of educational debt—there are options to reduce the cost of veterinary education if you look for them.

What challenges have you faced while practicing veterinary medicine?
Veterinarians are hardworking people with high expectations of themselves, and I am no exception. I have found it important to learn how to make time for non-veterinary pursuits such as family time, exercise, and hobbies. You have to take care of yourself, mind and body.

GEOGRAPHICAL LISTING OF AAVMC INSTITUTIONAL (AVMA/COE ACCREDITED) VETERINARY SCHOOLS AND DIRECTORY OF ADMISSIONS OFFICES

Atlantic Veterinary College at the
University of Prince Edward
Island (CANADA)
Registrar's Office
550 University Avenue
Charlottetown PEI C1A 4P3
Canada

Auburn University (USA)
Office for Academic Affairs
College of Veterinary Medicine
217 Goodwin/Overton
Auburn, AL 36849-5536

Colorado State University (USA)
College of Veterinary Medicine and
Biomedical Sciences
1601 Campus Delivery – Office of
the Dean
Fort Collins, CO 80523-1601

Cornell University (USA)
Office of Student & Academic Services
College of Veterinary Medicine
S2-009 Schurman Hall
Ithaca, NY 14853-6401

Iowa State University (USA)
Office of Admissions
College of Veterinary Medicine
2270 Veterinary Medicine
P.O. Box 3020
Ames, IA 50010-3020

Kansas State University (USA)
Office of Admissions
College of Veterinary Medicine
101 Trotter Hall
Manhattan, KS 66506-5601

Lincoln Memorial University (USA)
College of Veterinary Medicine
6965 Cumberland Gap Pkway
Harrogate, TN 37752

Louisiana State University (USA)
Office of Student and Academic Affairs
School of Veterinary Medicine
Skip Bertman Drive
Baton Rouge, LA 70803

Massey University Veterinary School
(AUSTRALIA)
International Student Affairs
Undergraduate Office
IVABS
Private Bag 11-222
Palmerston North 4442
New Zealand

Michigan State University (USA)
Office of Admissions
College of Veterinary Medicine
784 Wilson Road
F-110 Veterinary Medical Center
East Lansing, MI 48824

Midwestern University (USA)
College of Veterinary Medicine
19555 North 59th Avenue
Glendale, AZ 85308

Mississippi State University (USA)
Office of Student Admissions
College of Veterinary Medicine
P.O. Box 6100
Mississippi State, MS 39762

Murdoch University
(AUSTRALIA)
Murdoch International
South Street
Murdoch 6150
Western Australia

North Carolina State University (USA)
Student Services Office
College of Veterinary Medicine
1060 William Moore Drive, Box 8401
Raleigh, NC 27607

The Ohio State University (USA)
Office of Student Affairs
College of Veterinary Medicine
Suite 127 Veterinary Medicine
Academic Building
1900 Coffey Road
Columbus, OH 43210-1089

Oklahoma State University (USA)
Office of Admissions
112 McElroy Hall
Center for Veterinary Health
Sciences
College of Veterinary Medicine
Stillwater, OK 74078-2003

Oregon State University (USA)
Office of the Dean
Attention: Admissions
College of Veterinary Medicine
200 Magruder Hall
Corvallis, OR 97331-4801

Purdue University (USA)
Student Services Center
College of Veterinary Medicine
625 Harrison Street
West Lafayette, IN 47907-2026

Ross University School of Veterinary
Medicine (WEST INDIES)
Office of Admissions
630 US HWY 1
North Brunswick, NJ 08902

Royal Veterinary College
(UNITED KINGDOM)
Head of Admissions
Royal College Street
London NW1 0TU
United Kingdom

St. George's University
    (WEST INDIES)
Office of Admission
c/o The North American
    Correspondent
University Support Services, LLC
3500 Sunrise Highway
Building 300
Great River, NY 11739

Texas A & M University (USA)
Office of the Dean
College of Veterinary Medicine
    & Biomedical Sciences
College Station, TX 77843-4461

Tufts University (USA)
Office of Admissions
Cummings School of Veterinary
    Medicine
200 Westboro Road
North Grafton, MA 01536

Tuskegee University (USA)
Office of Admissions and
    Recruitment
School of Veterinary Medicine
100 Dr. Frederick Patterson Hall
Tuskegee, AL 36088

Universidad Nacional Autónoma
    de México (MEXICO)
Office of Undergraduate
    Studies (Division de Estudios
    Profesionales)
College of Veterinary Medicine
    (FMVZ)
Av. Universidad 3000
Circuito Interior
Delegacion Coyoacan
Mexico D.F. 04510

Université de Montréal (CANADA)
Service des Admissions
C.P. 6205
Succursale Centre-Ville
Montréal Québec H3C 3T5 Canada

University of Calgary (CANADA)
Admissions Office
Faculty of Veterinary Medicine
TRW 2D03
3280 Hospital Drive NW
Calgary, AB T2N 4Z6

University of California (USA)
School of Veterinary Medicine
Office of the Dean-Student
    Programs
One Shields Avenue
Davis, CA 95616

University College Dublin
    (IRELAND)
Veterinary Medicine Applications
UCD Admissions Office
Tierney Building
Belfield, Dublin 4
Ireland

University of Edinburgh
    (UNITED KINGDOM)
Admissions Office
Royal (Dick) School of Veterinary
    Studies
Easter Bush Veterinary Centre
Roslin EH25 9RG
Scotland

University of Florida (USA)
Admissions Office
College of Veterinary Medicine
P.O. Box 100125
Gainesville, FL 32610-0125

The University of Georgia (USA)
Admissions Department
Office for Academic Affairs
College of Veterinary Medicine
Athens, GA 30602-7372

University of Glasgow
    (UNITED KINGDOM)
Director of Admissions & Student
    Services Manager
College of Medicine, Veterinary and
    Life Sciences
School of Veterinary Medicine
    Undergraduate School
464 Bearsden Road
Glasgow G61 1QH

University of Guelph (CANADA)
Admissions Services
University Centre, Level 3
Guelph Ontario N 1G 2W 1
Canada

University of Illinois (USA)
College of Veterinary Medicine
Office of Academic and Student
    Affairs
2001 South Lincoln Avenue,
    Room 2271g
Urbana, IL 61802

University of Melbourne
    (AUSTRALIA)
Faculty of Veterinary Science
Corner Park Drive and
    Flemington Road
Parkville
Melbourne 3010
Victoria Australia

University of Minnesota (USA)
Office of Academic and Student Affairs
College of Veterinary Medicine
108 Pomeroy Center
1964 Fitch Ave.
St. Paul, MN 55108

University of Missouri-Columbia
    (USA)
Office of Academic Affairs
College of Veterinary Medicine
W203 Veterinary Medicine Building
Columbia, MO 65211

University of Pennsylvania (USA)
Admissions Office
School of Veterinary Medicine
3800 Spruce Street
Philadelphia, PA 19104-6044

The University of Queensland–
    Gatton Campus (AUSTRALIA)
School of Veterinary Science
Gatton, 4343
Queensland, Australia

University of Saskatchewan
   (CANADA)
Admissions Office
Western College of Veterinary
   Medicine
52 Campus Drive
Saskatoon Saskatchewan S7N 5B4
Canada

University of Sydney
   (AUSTRALIA)
Faculty of Veterinary Science
Sydney, NSW 2006
Australia

University of Tennessee (USA)
Admissions Office
College of Veterinary Medicine
2407 River Drive
Room A-104-C
Knoxville, TN 37996-4550

University of Wisconsin-Madison
   (USA)
Office of Academic Affairs
School of Veterinary Medicine
2015 Linden Drive
Madison, WI 53706-1102

Utrecht University
   (NETHERLANDS)
Office for International Cooperation
Faculty of Veterinary Medicine
Yalelaan 1
3584 CL Utrecht
The Netherlands

VetAgro Sup (FRANCE)
1, avenue Bourgelat
69280 Marcy l'Etoile
France

Virginia-Maryland College
   of Veterinary Medicine (USA)
Admissions Coordinator
Blacksburg, VA 24061

Washington State University (USA)
Office of Student Services
College of Veterinary Medicine
100 Grimes Way
P.O. Box 647012
Pullman, WA 99164-7012

Western University of Health
   Sciences (USA)
Office of Admissions
College of Veterinary Medicine
309 East 2nd Street
Pomona, CA 91766-1854

GEOGRAPHICAL LISTING OF AAVMC AFFILIATE (NON-AVMA/COE ACCREDITED) VETERINARY SCHOOLS AND DIRECTORY OF ADMISSIONS OFFICES

University of Adelaide
  (AUSTRALIA)
The School of Animal and
  Veterinary Science
Roseworthy Campus
Roseworthy SA 5371
Australia

Central Luzon State University
  (PHILIPPINES)
Science City of Munoz
Nueva Ecija 3120
Philippines

University of Copenhagen
  (DENMARK)
Office for International Cooperation
Faculty of Health and Medicine
Blegdamsvej 3B
DK-2200 Copenhagen N
Denmark

Seoul National University
  (SOUTH KOREA)
1 Gwanak-ro
Gwanak-gu, Seoul
South Korea

St. Matthew's University (USA)
Office of Admissions
12124 High Tech Avenue,
Suite 350
Orlando, Fl 32817

University of Tokyo (JAPAN)
Tokyo 113-8657
Japan

LISTING OF CONTRACTING STATES AND PROVINCES

Six Canadian provinces and 19 states in the United States have a veterinary school contract with one or more schools to provide access to veterinary medical education for their residents. The state or province, working through the contracting agency, usually agrees to pay a fee to help cover the cost of education for a certain number of places in each entering class. Residents from the contract states then compete with each other for those positions.

Some states contract with more than one school. For example, Arkansas contracts with 5 veterinary schools, and North Dakota contracts with 6 schools. Connecticut, Rhode Island, Vermont, Nebraska, and the District of Columbia presently have no contracts, so all candidates from these places apply as nonresidents to veterinary schools of their choice.

The educational agreements between contracting agencies and veterinary schools differ. Under some contract arrangements, students pay in-state tuition; in others, they pay nonresident tuition. Some contract states require students to repay all or part of the subsidy that the state provided; others require veterinary graduates to return to practice in the state for a period of time. Applicants should be aware of their obligation to the state before agreeing to participate in a contract program.

Following is a list of states and provinces that have educational agreements with schools of veterinary medicine.

UNITED STATES

ARIZONA

Contracts through WICHE* with University of California, Colorado State University, Oregon State University, and Washington State University.

ARKANSAS

Contracts in past with Louisiana State University, University of Missouri, and Oklahoma State University. Contracts not all completed at time of printing; may be some changes.

CONNECTICUT

Contracts with Iowa State University.

DELAWARE

Contracts with Oklahoma State University and the University of Georgia.

HAWAII

Contracts through WICHE* with University of California, Colorado State University, Oregon State University, and Washington State University.

IDAHO

Contracts with Washington State University.

KENTUCKY

Contracts with Auburn University and Tuskegee University.

MONTANA

Contracts through WICHE* with University of California, Colorado State University, Oregon State University, and Washington State University.

NEBRASKA

Formal education alliance with Iowa State University.

NEVADA

Contracts through WICHE* with University of California, Colorado State University, Oregon State University, and Washington State University.

NEW MEXICO

Contracts through WICHE* with University of California, Colorado State University, Oregon State University, and Washington State University.

NORTH DAKOTA

Contracts with Iowa State University, University of Minnesota, and Kansas State University. Contracts through WICHE* with the University of California, Colorado State University, Oregon State University, and Washington State University.

SOUTH CAROLINA

Contracts with University of Georgia , Mississippi State University, and Tuskegee University.

SOUTH DAKOTA

Reciprocity with University of Minnesota. Contracts with Iowa State University.

UTAH

Contracts through WICHE* with University of California, Colorado State University, and Oregon State University. Contracts with Washington State University.

* WICHE = Western Interstate Commission for Higher Education (offices in Boulder, Colorado)

WEST VIRGINIA

Contracts with Tuskegee University, Mississippi State University, Auburn University, and Virginia-Maryland College of Veterinary Medicine.

WYOMING

Contracts through WICHE* with the University of California, Colorado State University, Oregon State University, and Washington State University.

CANADA

ALBERTA

Contracts with University of Saskatchewan and University of Calgary.

BRITISH COLUMBIA

Contracts with University of Saskatchewan.

MANITOBA

Contracts with University of Saskatchewan.

NEW BRUNSWICK

Contracts with Atlantic Veterinary College at the University of Prince Edward Island and Université de Montréal.

NEWFOUNDLAND

Contracts with Atlantic Veterinary College at the University of Prince Edward Island.

NOVA SCOTIA

Contracts with Atlantic Veterinary College at the University of Prince Edward Island.

* WICHE = Western Interstate Commission for Higher Education (offices in Boulder, Colorado)

PROGRAMS FOR MULTICULTURAL OR DISADVANTAGED STUDENTS

The Association of American Veterinary Medical Colleges affirms the value of diversity within the veterinary medical profession. The membership is committed to incorporating that belief into their actions by advocating for the recruitment and retention of underrepresented persons as students and faculty, and ultimately fostering their success in the profession of veterinary medicine. The Association believes that through these actions, society and the profession will be well served.

Many schools have programs designed to facilitate entry into, and retention by, veterinary programs nationwide. These programs are directed at several levels, from high-school students to the student who has already been accepted by a veterinary college. Most of these programs will accept students from every state, regardless of the school(s) to which an individual might eventually apply or attend.

Following is an alphabetical list of schools by state and a short explanation of their programs:

UNIVERSITY OF CALIFORNIA

Program: Summer Enrichment Program

Description: a 6-week summer program. The purpose of this program is to increase the academic preparedness of disadvantaged students through science-based learning skills development, clinical education, individual advising, and student development.

Eligibility: Educationally and/or economically disadvantaged. Must have completed at least one year of college with a minimum science GPA of 2.8 and demonstrated interest in veterinary medicine.

Program dates: July–August.

Contact: Office of the Dean–Student Programs, School of Veterinary Medicine, University of California, One Shields Avenue, Davis CA 95616; telephone: (530) 752-1383.

Sponsorship: School of Veterinary Medicine, University of California-Davis.

COLORADO STATE UNIVERSITY

Program: Vet Prep

Description: a one-year academic program that serves as a bridge to the professional veterinary medical program for disadvantaged (cultural, social, economic) applicants who ranked high but were denied admission during the current admissions process. Limited to 10 students who upon successful completion are

guaranteed admission to the veterinary program. Candidates are selected from the current regular admissions applicant pool.

Eligibility: disadvantaged students.

Contact: College of Veterinary Medicine and Biomedical Sciences, W102 Anatomy, Colorado State University, Fort Collins CO 80523; telephone: (970) 491-7051; email: DVMAdmissions@colostate.edu.

Sponsorship: College of Veterinary Medicine and Biomedical Sciences, Colorado State University.

Program: Vet Start

Description: an 8-year undergraduate and professional program for students who enter Colorado State from high school resulting in a bachelor's and a professional degree. Undergraduate and professional program scholarships are provided, and admission to the professional veterinary medical program is guaranteed upon successful completion of the undergraduate requirements. Mentoring, support services, and summer jobs are available to participants.

Eligibility: students who have a disadvantaged background (economic, cultural, or social) will be given special consideration. Students must be high-school graduates with fewer than 15 semester credits of college coursework post high school graduation. Selection is competitive. There are 5 positions per year for incoming freshman undergraduate students.

Program dates: begins fall semester; applications available online early December; application deadline typically March 1.

Contact: College of Veterinary Medicine and Biomedical Sciences, Campus Delivery 1601, Colorado State University, Fort Collins CO 80523-1601; telephone: (970) 491-7051; email: ken.blehm@colostate.edu.

Sponsorship: College of Veterinary Medicine and Biomedical Sciences, Colorado State University.

CORNELL UNIVERSITY

Program: State University of New York Graduate Underrepresented Minority Fellowships

Description: all matriculating underrepresented minorities are eligible (not restricted by state residency).

Contact: Director of Student Financial Planning, Office of Student & Academic Services, College of Veterinary Medicine, Cornell University, S2-009 Schurman Hall, Ithaca NY 14853-6401; telephone: (607) 253-3766; website: www.vet.cornell.edu/financialaid.

MICHIGAN STATE UNIVERSITY

Program: Vetward Bound Program

Description: Vetward Bound offers different levels of programming, each with its own eligibility requirements. The program provides a review of basic science content, research and/or clinical experience, preparation for the GRE, veterinary experience, food and fiber animal experience, study strategy development, and field experiences. Level placement is determined by program staff and is based on educational background.

Eligibility: Economically and educationally disadvantaged first year undergraduate students through pre-matriculants into the professional degree program. Students selected to participate will meet HHS Health Careers Opportunity Program guidelines and Federal thresholds. An individual will be determined to be disadvantaged if he or she comes from a background that has inhibited the individual from obtaining the knowledge, skills, and abilities required to enroll in and graduate from a health professions school or comes from a family with an annual income below a level based on low income thresholds according to family size published by the Bureau of the Census, adjusted annually for changes in the Consumer Price Index, and adjusted by the Secretary for use in health professions programs.

Program dates: June–July.

Contact: Vetward Bound Coordinator, College of Veterinary Medicine, 784 Wilson Road, F-110 Veterinary Medical Center, Michigan State University, East Lansing MI 48824; telephone: (517) 355-6521; email: vetbound@cvm.msu.edu.

MISSISSIPPI STATE UNIVERSITY

Program: Board of Trustees of State Institutions of Higher Learning Veterinary Medicine Minority Loan/Scholarship Program

Description: a financial assistance program for Mississippi residents who are underrepresented minorities. The loan to service obligation is one year for each year of scholarship assistance, not to exceed four years.

Contact: Susan Eckels, Program Administrator, Mississippi Institutions of Higher Learning, 3825 Ridgewood Road, Jackson MS 39211-6453; telephone: (800) 327-2980.

NORTH CAROLINA STATE UNIVERSITY

Program: UNC Campus Scholarship Program—Graduate Student Component

Description: UNC General Administration funds this program. Eligibility is limited to new or continuing full-time doctoral students who have financial need and who are residents of North Carolina as of the beginning of the award period (as determined under the *Manual to Assist the Public Higher Education Institutions of N.C. in the Matter of Student Resident Classification for Tuition Purposes*). Individuals who have been accepted to a master's degree program in a department offering the doctoral degree and who intend, and will be eligible, to pursue doctoral studies at NC State after completion of the requirements for the master's degree are also eligible. The program provides up to $3,000 annually for North Carolina residents.

Contact: Director of Diversity Affairs, College of Veterinary Medicine, North Carolina State University, 1060 William Moore Drive, Box 8401, Raleigh, NC 27607; telephone: (919) 513-6262; website: www.cvm.ncsu.edu.

Program: Diversity Graduate Assistant Grant

Description: Funded by the North Carolina State University Graduate School, recipients must be full-time, new or continuing students pursuing master's and doctoral degrees at North Carolina State University. The program provides up to $3,000 annually. Both resident and nonresident students are eligible to apply.

Contact: Director of Diversity Affairs, College of Veterinary Medicine, North Carolina State University, 1060 William Moore Drive, Box 8401, Raleigh, NC 27607; telephone: (919) 513-6262; website: www.cvm.ncsu.edu.

Note: North Carolina residents are encouraged to apply for both programs. However, the annual maximum award for these grant programs is a combined $3,000 (with an option of $500 in additional support for study in the summer). The grant is awarded on an annual basis. Awardees must reapply each year.

THE OHIO STATE UNIVERSITY

Program: Young Scholars Program

Description: this summer program is offered to seventh- through eleventh-grade students from Ohio. It provides hands-on science activities, academic enrichment exercises, and career exploration opportunities.

Eligibility: disadvantaged students recommended by their faculty.

Program dates: June to August each summer.

Sponsorship: the State of Ohio and The Ohio State University.

Program: Summer Research Opportunity Program

Description: this program is designed to promote the migration of minority undergraduate students into graduate research educational programs by providing them with summer research experiences. The student is provided with his or her individualized research problem by a faculty mentor and expected to carry that research through to publication.

Eligibility: the student must have completed 2 years of college work and have achieved at least a 2.50 cumulative GPA. The student must be an underrepresented minority or economically disadvantaged.

Contact: Graduate School, The Ohio State University, 230 North Oval Mall, Columbus OH 43210.

Sponsorship: the Big Ten Consortium for Institutional Studies.

PURDUE UNIVERSITY

Program: Access to Animal-Related Careers (A²RC)

Description: A²RC is a two-week, residential program offering hands-on experiences in multiple areas of veterinary medicine including swine production medicine, small animal medicine, and equine medicine. Also included are sessions on several specialty areas such as cardiology, emergency and critical care medicine, and radiology. The program is designed to expose participants to life as a first year DVM student. Mock admissions interviews are conducted and participants are given individual feedback.

Eligibility: A²RC is targeted to 2nd and 3rd year underrepresented minority undergraduate students at partner institutions enrolled in pre-veterinary studies.

Program dates: May 15-28, 2016.

Contact: Dr. Kauline Cipriani Davis, Director of Diversity Initiatives (cipriank@purdue.edu or 765 496-1940; website http://www.vet.purdue.edu/diversity/index.php)

UNIVERSITY OF TENNESSEE

Program: Veterinary Summer Experience for Tennessee High School Students

Description: The College of Veterinary Medicine offers an eight-week program that provides high school students an opportunity to gain experience working with veterinarians at a veterinary practice in their home towns for seven weeks during the summer. During the eighth week of this summer experience, students will be guests of the College of Veterinary Medicine on the campus of The University of Tennessee in Knoxville. Students will attend clinical rotations in the Equine, Farm Animal, Small Animal, and Avian and Exotic Animal (including zoo medicine) Hospitals in the Veterinary Medical Center. Students will also attend special educational functions related to veterinary medicine.

Eligibility: To qualify for this summer program, a student must be a Tennessee resident and be at least 16 years of age by June 1, be enrolled as a senior or junior in a Tennessee high school, and have earned a minimum 3.0 high school GPA. Applicants must also have an interest in veterinary medicine as a potential career. Preference will be given to applicants who will contribute greatly to the diversity of the summer program and, potentially, to the veterinary profession. Students receive a financial stipend for satisfactory performance in the eight-week program.

Program dates: Summer.

Contact: Dr. William Hill, The University of Tennessee, College of Veterinary Medicine, 2431 Joe Johnson Drive, 339 Ellington Plant Science, Knoxville TN 37996, telephone: (865) 974-5770. E-mail: wahill@utk.edu.

UNIVERSITY OF MINNESOTA

Program: Veterinary Leadership in Early Admissions for Diversity (VetLEAD)

Description: VetLEAD creates a pathway into the DVM program for high-ability students at underrepresented serving partner schools, including Florida Agricultural and Mechanical University (FAMU).

Eligibility: Any high-achieving student enrolled in the Animal Science program at FAMU may apply for an early admissions decision at the end of their sophomore year of undergraduate studies. Eligible students have past experience working or volunteering in a veterinary related setting, a FAMU cumulative GPA of 3.4 with coursework consistent with required prerequisite courses, and strong letters of references.

Contact: Karen Nelson, Director of Admissions, dvminfo@umn.edu

TUSKEGEE UNIVERSITY

Program: Summer Enrichment and Reinforcement Program (SERP)

Description: this 8-week preadmission program is designed to provide academic enrichment through effective learning strategies and mentorship to facilitate the entry of "at risk" students into the veterinary program and successful transition through the professional curriculum.

Eligibility: participation is targeted to minority and disadvantaged students who have completed at least 3 years of college and all Pre-Veterinary prerequisites. Participation is restricted to persons who have applied to the DVM program in the College of Veterinary Medicine, Nursing, and Allied Health and who have been recommended by the Veterinary Admissions Committee for evaluation to the program.

Program dates: the summer before fall semester.

Contact: Associate Dean for Academic Affairs, College of Veterinary Medicine, Nursing and Allied Health, Tuskegee University, Tuskegee, AL 36088.

Sponsorship: this program is sponsored by a grant from the U.S. Department of Health and Human Services.

Program: Veterinary Science Training, Education and Preparation Institutes for Minority Students (Vet-Step I and II)

Description: Consists of 2 one-week programs designed to encourage high achieving minority students to consider veterinary medicine as a career choice. The program focus on progressive learning skills in reading comprehension, study skills, time-management, note-taking, medical vocabulary, etc.

Eligibility: Vet-Step I accepts 30 students from grades 9 and 10; Vet-Step II accepts students from Vet-Step I and from grade 12. Minority high school honor students interested in the biomedical sciences are strongly encouraged to apply.

Contact: Coordinator, Vet-Step Program, College of Veterinary Medicine, Nursing, and Allied Health, Tuskegee University, Tuskegee AL 36088, (334) 727-8309.

Sponsorship: U.S. Department of Health and Human Services.

VIRGINIA-MARYLAND COLLEGE OF VETERINARY MEDICINE

Program: Multicultural Academic Opportunities Program

Description: a 10-week program providing opportunities to conduct scientific research; participate in clinical rotations within the veterinary teaching hospital; improve leadership, public speaking, and self-marketing skills; attend GRE preparatory classes; and learn about admission into graduate / professional school.

Contact: Admissions Office at Blacksburg campus.

Program: Summer Research Apprenticeship Program —College Park

Description: a summer research program providing research experience to veterinary and Pre-Veterinary students from diverse backgrounds, including economic hardship and underrepresented racial/ethnic groups. Projects may include assisting in the planning, preparation, and data collection for controlled experiments, clinical trials, or epidemiological investigations; researching disease processes; and performing literature searches.

Contact: Admissions Office at College Park campus.

Scholarship Opportunities: a limited number of scholarships are available to assist minority DVM students.

WASHINGTON STATE UNIVERSITY

Program: Short-Term Research Training Program for Veterinary Students

Description: a 3-month summer program designed to promote interest in research by veterinary students. Emphasis is on a hands-on research project supervised by a faculty member with a research program. Stipends are provided.

Eligibility: WSU veterinary students or ethnic minority veterinary students from other U.S. colleges of veterinary medicine.

Program dates: 3 months in the summer dependent upon the summer vacation of the WSU College of Veterinary Medicine in which the veterinary student is enrolled.

Contact: Department of Veterinary Microbiology and Pathology, Washington State University, Pullman WA 99164-7040.

Sponsorship: The National Center for Research Resources.

UNIVERSITY OF WISCONSIN

Program: Pre-College Enrollment Opportunity Program for Learning Excellence (PEOPLE)

Description: this program began in the summer of 1999 as a partnership between the Milwaukee Public Schools and the UW-Madison with a group of students who had just completed the ninth grade. New classes will be added each year, expanding to Madison area schools. The program is designed with a precollege track and a bridge program to undergraduate work and continues through a student's undergraduate career at University of Wisconsin-Madison. The main purposes are to promote academic preparation, increase enrollment in postsecondary institutions, and improve retention and graduation rates of minority and disadvantaged students.

Eligibility: students of one or more of the following ethnic heritages: African American, American Indian, Asian American, Hispanic/Latino. Other eligibility factors include economic disadvantage and current enrollment in or commitment to a college preparatory curriculum track.

Program dates: June–July summer residential programs and year-round nonresidential programs.

Contact: PEOPLE Program, 1305 Linden Drive, University of Wisconsin- Madison, Madison, WI 53706.

FINANCIAL AID INFORMATION

Financing your veterinary medical education requires careful planning, good money management skills, and a willingness to make short-term sacrifices to achieve long-range goals.

Many of you will apply for and receive some type of financial assistance during your undergraduate education. This will help you become somewhat familiar with the process, and to know that the rules and regulations governing programs can and do change periodically.

> Don't live the lifestyle of a DVM until you have completed your education. Get in the habit of being thrifty.

As a professional student, you will be entering a partnership with the financial aid office, which will require you to complete the appropriate financial aid forms accurately, meet required deadlines, and submit any additional information that may be requested. In return, the financial aid office will determine your aid eligibility and make awards based on the available programs. Your financial aid eligibility takes into account the cost of your education minus any other available resources. Amounts of assistance and the school policies for awarding assistance vary from one veterinary medical school to another and from year to year.

Any questions or concerns that you may have about this topic need to be directed to each of the appropriate financial aid offices to ensure that you receive accurate information and guidance.

FINANCING YOUR VETERINARY MEDICAL EDUCATION

Your education is one of the biggest investments you will make in your lifetime, and one of your most important goals should be to maximize the return on all of your investments. To reach this goal, you must take an active role in managing your financial resources. You need to understand and implement good financial practices. To get you started, here are some good financial habits you should adopt:

- Do not use credit cards to extend your lifestyle. Deciding not to use credit cards except in emergencies is one of the most important decisions you can make, and one that will reduce your stress while you are pursuing your education.
- Budget your money just as carefully as you budget your time. Contact a financial aid administrator to help you set up a budget that will be easy to follow.
- Distinguish between wants and needs. Before you make any purchase, you should ask yourself, "Do I need this, or do I want it?"
- Be a well-informed borrower. If you have not previously taken an active role in understanding the differences between various student loan programs, now is the time to do it. You need to know these differences in order to avoid high-interest loans and to borrow wisely.
- Borrow the minimum amount necessary in order to maximize the return on your educational investment.
- Be thrifty. Live as cheaply as you can. Remember, you are a student. You'll enjoy a more comfortable lifestyle once you are a DVM.
- Pay any interest that accrues on student loans if you can afford to do so, rather than let the interest accrue and capitalize. Any amount you pay while you're a student will save you money once you enter repayment.

What is the most important piece of advice for making the most of your educational investment? Don't live the lifestyle of a DVM until you have completed your education. Get in the habit of being thrifty. If you live like a DVM while you are in school, you may have to live like a student when you are a DVM.

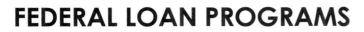

FEDERAL LOAN PROGRAMS

Please note that subsidized loans are not available beginning fall 2012.

	William D. Ford Unsubsidized Stafford Loan	Perkins Loan	Health Professions Student Loan	Loan for Disadvantaged Students	Grad Plus Loans for Graduate/ Professional Students
Lender	Federal Loan Program	Federal Loan Program	Federal Loan Program	Federal Loan Program	Federal Loan Program
Financial Need	No	Yes	Yes	Yes	No
Citizenship Requirement	U.S. Citizen, U.S. National, or U.S. Permanent Resident	U.S. Citizen, U.S. National, or U.S. Permanent Resident	U.S. Citizen, U.S. National, or U.S. Permanent Resident	U.S. Citizen, U.S. National, or U.S. Permanent Resident	U.S. Citizen, U.S. National, or U.S. Permanent Resident
Borrowing Limits	Cost of attendance minus other aid; $189,125 aggregate undergraduate and graduate	$6,000/year; $40,000 aggregate undergraduate and graduate	Cost of attendance at participating school	Federal Loan Programs	Cost of attendance minus other aid
Interest Rate	Fixed; capped at 6.8%	5%	5%	5%	7%
Interest Accrues While Enrolled in School	Yes	No	No	No	Yes
Deferments	Yes	Yes	Yes	Yes	Yes
Grace Period	Yes	Yes	Yes	Yes	No

A GUIDE TO PREPARING FOR VETERINARY SCHOOL

Maybe you already know that you have a strong interest in veterinary medicine, but you don't know where to start. It's never too early to begin preparing. Below are a few guidelines to help you plan your coursework and get in touch with mentors and other professionals who can help you along the way.

HIGH SCHOOL STUDENTS

- Take science and math classes, including chemistry, biology, and algebra. If available, take Advanced Placement (AP) coursework. Note, AP courses may not always satisfy vet college prerequisite coursework, but they will give you the highest level of preparation. Consult with the vet colleges to understand if AP credit in high school will satisfy a prerequisite course requirement.
- Talk to people in the field. Call local veterinarians or contact a veterinary society in your city or town to find people who can help answer your questions.
- Gain animal experiences. These will give you a good understanding of working with animals and excellent references when you seek a volunteer experience or internship with a veterinarian. Examples include volunteering at a humane society, cleaning stables and grooming horses, doing an internship at a zoo, volunteering at a nature or wildlife center, or getting involved with 4-H, just to name a few.
- Visit veterinary college websites and perhaps make a visit during one of their admissions presentations or during an open house. The more you know early on, the better prepared you will be.
- Get on the veterinary college's mailing lists for admissions updates and invitations to programs.

COLLEGE YEAR 1

Fall semester
- Obtain a copy of the *AAVMC Veterinary Medical School Admission Requirements* (*VMSAR*) to review the veterinary schools' requirements with your advisor.
- Meet with an advisor and plan coursework. Take the list of prerequisite courses on the AAVMC website or in *VMSAR* for planning purposes. Not all vet colleges require the exact same courses, but most will want courses in the areas of biology, chemistry, and physics. That's a good place to start until you narrow down your list of vet colleges to apply to.
- Start working on the prerequisite coursework. Most vet colleges require quite a few biology and chemistry courses. Starting out right away in these introductory courses will allow you to move forward quickly.

Spring semester
- Think about summer volunteer or employment opportunities in veterinary medicine, such as shadowing a veterinarian or volunteering in an animal shelter.
- Continue working on the introductory courses and register for the fall semester.
- Research preveterinary enrichment programs at ExploreHealthCareers.org. Preveterinary enrichment programs can help you decide if a career in veterinary medicine is a good fit and help prepare you for the application process.

Summer
- Complete an internship or volunteer program.
- Attend summer school, if necessary. Note, many vet colleges prefer the prerequisite coursework be taken in a full-time load during the academic year. If possible, take general education or major courses during the summer.

COLLEGE YEAR 2

Fall semester
- Meet with your advisor to discuss your progress.
- Attend preveterinary activities.
- Join your school's preveterinary society, if one is available.
- Continue working on prerequisite coursework.
- Explore community service opportunities through your school (they don't necessarily need to be animal-related). If possible, continue activities throughout undergraduate career.

Spring semester
- Look into paid or volunteer veterinary-related research opportunities.
- Complete second semester coursework and register for the fall.

Summer
- Complete a summer research or volunteer veterinary-related program.
- Attend summer school, if necessary.
- Prepare for the Graduate Record Examination (GRE).

- Visit veterinary colleges. Meet with someone from the admissions office or attend an admissions presentation and take a tour.

COLLEGE YEAR 3

Fall semester

- Meet with your preveterinary advisor.
- Discuss veterinary schools.
- Register for spring semester.
- Visit the AAVMC's website (www.aavmc.org) to learn about applying to veterinary schools.
- Place your order for the *AAVMC Veterinary Medical School Admission Requirements.*
- Research schools.

Spring semester

- Identify individuals (veterinarian, faculty member or advisor, supervisor of animal experiences, research faculty) to write letters of recommendation.
- Take the GRE during late spring or early summer.
- Prepare to submit your vet school applications.
- Register for the fall semester.
- Schedule a volunteer or paid veterinary medicine-related activity.

Summer

- Take the GRE if you have not done so already.
- Budget time and finances appropriately to attend interviews.
- Participate in a volunteer or paid opportunity.
- Attend summer school, if necessary.
- Work on and submit your applications. Most vet colleges have a supplemental application, so be very careful to meet **all deadlines** for the VMCAS application, supplemental application, and getting in supporting documentation and letters.

COLLEGE YEAR 4

Fall semester

- Meet with your advisor.
- Attend interviews with schools.
- Notification of acceptances begins December 1.

Spring semester

- Apply for federal financial aid.
- April 15 deadline to let the vet colleges where you have been admitted know your decision.

Summer

- Attend school's orientation.
- Prepare to relocate, if necessary.

VETERINARY MEDICAL COLLEGE APPLICATION SERVICE (VMCAS)

The Veterinary Medical College Application Service is a centralized application service sponsored by the Association of American Veterinary Medical Colleges. Applicants use VMCAS to apply to most of the AVMA-accredited colleges in the United States and abroad.

VMCAS collects, processes, and ships application materials to veterinary colleges designated by the applicant, and responds to applicant inquiries about the application process. This service is the data collection, processing, and distribution component of the admission process for colleges participating in VMCAS. VMCAS, however, does not take part in the admissions selection process.

Twenty-nine (29) of the thirty (30) U.S. veterinary institutions participate in VMCAS, along with two (2) Canadian, two (2) Scottish, one (1) English, one (1) Irish, one (1) Australian, and one (1) New Zealand veterinary institutions. Application material deadlines, prerequisite courses, and other aspects of the admissions process differ from school to school. Applicants are responsible for being informed of all instructions provided by VMCAS and the associated member colleges. Questions about using VMCAS should be directed to the VMCAS Student and Advisor Hotline.

APPLICATION CYCLE TIMELINE

VMCAS launch: May 11, 2017
VMCAS Application Deadline: September 15, 2017, 12 Midnight Eastern Time
AAVMC Acceptance Deadline: April 16, 2018
Please be sure to verify individual school deadlines

KEY ONLINE RESOURCES

General Information Chart

A one-stop comparison of school info such as location, tuition, seat availability, etc.
http://aavmc.org/data/files/vmcas/geninfochart.pdf

Prerequisite Comparison Chart

A course requirement comparison chart of all AAVMC member schools.
http://aavmc.org/data/files/vmcas/prereqchart.pdf

Fee Structure

VMCAS fees broken down by number of designations.
http://aavmc.org/Applicant-Responsibilities/Fees.aspx

Evaluation Requirements

Individual recommendation requirements by school.
www.aavmc.org/Applicant-Responsibilities/Evaluations.aspx

Supplemental Applications

Additional applications required by some schools. http://aavmc.org/College-Specific-Requirements/College-Specific-Requirements_College-Specifications.aspx

VMCAS

655 K Street, NW Suite 725
Washington, DC 20001
Telephone: (617) 612-2884
Fax: (617) 612-2051
vmcasinfo@vmcas.org
www.aavmc.org

VETERINARY MEDICAL SCHOOLS IN THE **UNITED STATES**

AVMA/COE Accredited

AUBURN UNIVERSITY

Email Address: admissions@vetmed.auburn.edu
Website: http://www.vetmed.auburn.edu

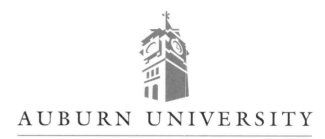

AUBURN UNIVERSITY

COLLEGE OF
VETERINARY MEDICINE

SCHOOL DESCRIPTION

The College of Veterinary Medicine at Auburn University is located in south central Alabama off Interstate 85 between Montgomery and Atlanta. The college is known for its friendly small-campus atmosphere.

Veterinary medicine began as a department at Auburn in 1892 and became a college in 1907. Today it is situated on 330 acres one mile from the main Auburn campus that serves more than 28,000 students. In addition, the college has a 700-acre research farm five miles from its campus. The college is fully accredited by the American Veterinary Medical Association.

> Students have the opportunity to work with more than 100 nationally and internationally recognized faculty.

APPLICATION INFORMATION

For specific application information (availability, deadlines, fees, and VMCAS participation), please refer to the contact information listed above.

Residency implications: 41 Alabama residents, 38 Kentucky residents, and 41 non-contract non-resident students.

Required undergraduate GPA: Alabama and Kentucky residents must have a minimum grade point average of 2.50 on a 4.00 scale. Applicants not classified as Alabama or Kentucky residents must have a minimum grade point average of 3.00 on a 4.00 scale. A grade of C-minus or better must be earned for any required course. The mean grade point average of the most recent entering class was 3.60.

AP credit policy: must appear on official college transcripts and be equivalent to the appropriate college-level coursework.

Course completion deadline: prerequisite courses must be completed by June 15 prior to matriculation.

Standardized examinations: Graduate Record Examination (GRE®), general test, is required. The exam must have been taken within the previous 5 calendar years, and must be received no later than September 15 of the year of application, therefore you should test no later than September 1.

GRE Code: 1005

ADDITIONAL REQUIREMENTS AND CONSIDERATIONS

A minimum of 500 hours of veterinary experience in addition to other animal experience

Recommendations (3 required)
Academic advisor or faculty member
Employer
Veterinarian

Extracurricular and community service activities

Narrative statement of purpose

SUMMARY OF ADMISSION PROCEDURES

VMCAS application deadline: Friday, September 15, 2017 at 12 Midnight Eastern Time

Date interviews are held: Non-contract, non-resident February; Alabama and Kentucky residents March

Date acceptances mailed: Within 12 days following interviews

PREREQUISITES FOR ADMISSION

Course Requirements	Number of Semester Hours
Written composition#	6
* Literature#	3
Fine Arts#	3
Humanities/fine arts elective#	6
* History#	3
Social/behavioral science electives#	9
Mathematics—precalculus with trigonometry#	3
Biology I with lab	4
Biology II with lab	4
Cell Biology	3
Fundamentals of chemistry with lab	8
Organic chemistry 1 with lab; Organic chemistry 2	6
Physics I	4
Biochemistry	3
Science electives**	6
## Animal Nutrition	3

* Students must complete a 6-semester-hour sequence either in literature or in history.

** Science electives must be two of the following: genetics, microbiology, physics II, comparative anatomy, histology, reproductive physiology, mammalian or animal physiology, parasitology, embryology, or immunology.

These requirements will be waived if the student has a bachelor's degree.

Will accept web based or correspondence course.

School begins: August

Deposit (to hold place in class): none required

Deferments: not considered

Transfer Students: Auburn does not take transfer students

International Students: not considered for admission

Evaluation criteria: Auburn University has a three-part admission procedure: an objective evaluation of academic credentials; a subjective review of personal credentials and experience under veterinary supervision; and a personal interview.

2016–2017 ADMISSIONS SUMMARY

Number of Applicants
Resident: 86
Contract*: 78
Non-resident: 790
Total: 954

Number of New Entrants
Resident: 41
Contract*: 38
Non-resident: 41
Total: 120

ESTIMATED TUITION

Tuition and fees
Resident: $18,696
Non-resident: $44,840
Contract*: $18,696

* For further information, see the listing of contracting states and provinces (see pg. 12).

** Please be aware that the estimated cost of attendance is higher for the third academic year when a summer semester is required because of the continuous year of clinical training.

ENTRANCE REQUIREMENTS

Admitted students fall into three categories: residents of Alabama, residents of Kentucky admitted by contract through the Southern Regional Education Board

(SREB), or at-large residents (non-Alabama and non-contract students).

Kentucky students must verify their residency status with their Kentucky pre-vet advisor before September 15. They may contact the Kentucky Council on Postsecondary Education for additional information.

Resident/contract applicants must be a documented resident of Alabama or Kentucky.

ADDITIONAL INFORMATION

Application Deadline: 9/15/2017

UNIVERSITY OF CALIFORNIA

Email Address: admissions@vetmed.ucdavis.edu
Website: http://www.vetmed.ucdavis.edu

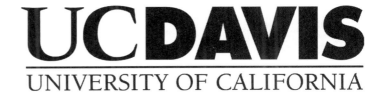

SCHOOL DESCRIPTION

The University of California, Davis (UC Davis) campus is one of 10 campuses of the University of California system. It is the largest campus, with 5,300 acres. The Davis campus is located in Yolo County in the Central Valley of Northern California. Davis is situated 11 miles west of Sacramento, 385 miles north of Los Angeles, and 72 miles northeast of San Francisco. Davis is surrounded by open space, including some of the most productive agricultural land in the state. The terrain is flat and the City of Davis is a friendly college town that cares about sustainability and welcoming newcomers. Ranked as one of the best towns to live in in the nation, Davis is also considered the most bike-friendly city in the nation. The Central Valley climate can be described as Mediterranean. The mild temperate climate means enjoyment of outdoors all year long. During the hot, dry, sunny summers, temperatures on some days can exceed 100 degrees F; however, more often summer temperatures are in the low 90s. Spring and fall has some of the most pleasant weather in the state. Winters in Davis are usually mild. UC Davis is an outstanding research and training institution with over 35,000 undergraduate, graduate and professional students. The Davis campus has four undergraduate colleges, graduate studies in all schools and colleges, and six professional programs carried out in the schools of Education, Law, Management, Medicine, Nursing, and Veterinary Medicine.

> UC Davis is an outstanding research and training institution with over 35,000 students.

Since 1948 the School of Veterinary Medicine serves the people of California by providing educational, research, clinical service, and public service programs of the highest quality to advance the health and care of animals, the public and the environment. School of Veterinary Medicine faculty members have earned a reputation for their broad expertise and shared commitment to solving some of society's most persistent health problems. The school's impact is evident in the accomplishments of clinicians who have developed novel treatments and basic scientists who continue to make major discoveries in animal, human and environmental health. We address the health of all animals, including livestock, poultry, companion animals, captive and free-ranging wildlife, exotic animals, birds, aquatic mammals and fish, and animals used in biological and medical research. Our expertise also encompasses related human health concerns.

To carry out this mission, we focus on students in our professional Doctor of Veterinary Medicine program, Master of Preventive Veterinary Medicine program, graduate clinical residency program and graduate academic MS and PhD programs. The school is fully committed to recruiting students with diverse backgrounds.

The School of Veterinary Medicine is home of the William R. Pritchard Veterinary Medical Teaching Hospital, Veterinary Medicine Teaching and Research Center, California Animal Health and Food Safety Laboratory, UC Veterinary Medical Center-San Diego and Centers of Excellence-fostering research, teaching and service focused on species interests and multidisciplinary themes. There are many other centers and innovative programs at UC Davis. Our statewide mission includes 28 research and clinical programs including continuing education; extension; and community outreach.

APPLICATION INFORMATION

For specific application information (availability, deadlines, fees, and VMCAS participation), please refer to our website at www.vetmed.ucdavis.edu.

Residency implications: A non-specified number of resident, nonresident, and WICHE applicants are accepted. International students are also considered for admission.

SUMMARY OF ADMISSION PROCEDURES

VMCAS application deadline: Friday, September 15, 2017 at 9 PM Pacific Time

Supplemental information is required. School will notify the applicant to set-up portal and complete supplemental information after application has been verified by VMCAS.

Date interviews are held: TBD (December or January)

Date admission notifications available in portal: TBD (January or February)

School begins: August

Deposit (to hold place in class): not required

Deferments: reviewed on a case-by-case basis for unexpected medical reasons or situations beyond control of applicant

EVALUATION CRITERIA

Cumulative Science GPA

Last (most recent) 45 semester/67.5 quarter units GPA

GRE Quantitative scores

VMCAS Electronic Letters of Recommendation (eLOR)

MMI Interview

ENTRANCE REQUIREMENTS

Required undergraduate GPA: a minimum grade point average of 2.50 on a 4.00 scale is required for all science courses completed and 2.50 on all courses cumulatively at time of application. Applicants admitted in fall 2016 had a mean cumulative GPA of 3.75 and a mean science GPA of 3.80.

AP credit policy: Credit must appear on official college transcript with course name and units awarded and must be equivalent to the prerequisite course being satisfied.

Is a Bachelor's Degree Required? yes

Is this an International School? no

ESTIMATED TUITION

Estimated Tuition Resident: $35,700

Estimated Tuition Contract: $47,945

Estimated Tuition Non-Resident: $47,945

AVAILABLE SEATS - 140

Resident: varied

Contract: varied

Non-Resident: varied

TEST REQUIREMENTS

Standardized examinations: Graduate Record Examination, general test is required. The acceptable GRE test dates for applicants entering 2018 are August 31, 2012 - August 31, 2017. Scores must be sent directly to VMCAS code 4804 by September 15, 2017.

VMCAS Participation: full

Accepts International Students? yes

ADDITIONAL INFORMATION

Dual-Degree Programs

Combined DVM/PhD graduate degree programs are available.

Visit our Veterinary Scientist Training Program information at www.vetmed.ucdavis.edu/vstp.

Application Deadline: 9/15/2017

COLORADO STATE UNIVERSITY

Email Address: dvmadmissions@colostate.edu
Website: http://csu-cvmbs.colostate.edu
/dvm-program/Pages/DVM-Program
-Entrance-Requirements.aspx

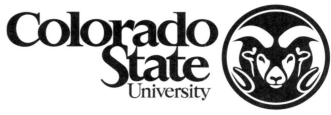

DOCTOR OF VETERINARY MEDICINE PROGRAM

SCHOOL DESCRIPTION

Colorado State University is located in Fort Collins, a city of about 150,000 in the eastern foothills of the Rocky Mountains about 65 miles north of Denver. Fort Collins has a pleasant climate and offers many cultural and recreational activities. Many of the state's ski areas lie within a short driving distance, making some of the best skiing in the world accessible. The nearby river canyons and mountain parks are beautiful scenic attractions and provide opportunities for hiking, fishing, photography, camping, and biking.

> Colorado State University is located in Fort Collins, a city of about 150,000 in the eastern foothills of the Rockies.

The College of Veterinary Medicine and Biomedical Sciences is nationally renowned for its programs in oncology, equine surgery and reproduction, and pain management. Our college is composed of eight major buildings that house the departments of biomedical sciences, environmental and radiological health sciences, and microbiology, immunology, and pathology.

The James L. Voss Veterinary Teaching Hospital, one of the world's largest and best equipped, houses the clinical sciences department. This department boasts a variety of unique units, including the internationally acclaimed Robert H. and Mary G. Flint Animal Cancer Center, Animal Population Health Institute, Integrated Livestock Management Program, and Gail Holmes Equine Orthopaedic Research Center. The hospital attracts a large caseload and offers students a wide variety of clinical experiences.

The uniquely designed Diagnostic Medicine Center houses the college's Veterinary Diagnostic Laboratory (VDL), the University's Extension Veterinarian, the Clinical Pathology Laboratory and the Animal Population Health Institute.

The VDL provides disease testing services to veterinarians, state/federal agencies, livestock owners and pet owners. The Clinical Pathology Laboratory provides services such as blood, fluid and urine analysis and cytology to identify diseases and illnesses in animals brought to the VTH or to veterinarians in the region. The Animal Population Health Institute encourages collaboration and information and expertise exchange in veterinary epidemiology among scientists at CSU, collaborating institutions and government agencies throughout the world.

Internationally known for its innovative curriculum, our veterinary program provides students with a four-year course of study in veterinary medicine leading to the Doctor of Veterinary Medicine degree. The first two years are conducted on the main campus and include comprehensive coverage of veterinary and biomedical sciences along with integrated hands-on and clinical experiences. During the second two years, students participate in animal care at the Veterinary Teaching Hospital through a series of specialty rotations. Students participate as team members in evaluating patients, meeting with clients, developing treatment plans, and providing hands-on care, all under the supervision of faculty clinicians.

PREREQUISITES FOR ADMISSION

Course Description	Number of Semester/Credits	Necessity
Biochemistry (that requires Org Chem)	3	Required
Genetics	3	Required
Physics (with a laboratory)	4	Required
Statistics	3	Required
Lab associated with a biology course	1	Required
Lab associated with a chemistry course	1	Required
English Composition	3	Required
Social sciences and humanities	12	Required
Electives	30	Required

APPLICATION INFORMATION

Application requirements: For your application to be reviewed by the Veterinary Admissions Committee, we must receive the following items before the deadline:

• VMCAS Application, three VMCAS eLORs, and Fee
• Colorado Supplemental Application (CSA) and Fee
• GRE Verbal, Quantitative, and Analytical (self-reported unofficial scores in the CSA)

SUMMARY OF ADMISSION PROCEDURES

Colorado Supplemental Application deadline: Friday, September 15, 2017 at 10 PM (MT). Fee: $80

VMCAS application deadline: Friday, September 15, 2017 at 12 Midnight (ET)

School begins: late August

Deposit: (to hold place in class) none required

Deferments: case-by-case basis for extenuating circumstances

EVALUATION CRITERIA

- Quality of academic program (course load, challenging curriculum, honors)
- GRE scores
- Veterinary/Animal/Research/Work Employment experience
- Extracurricular/Community/Leadership activities and achievements
- Essay
- Contribution to diversity, unique attributes, extenuating circumstances

• Letters of Reference, three VMCAS eLORs - veterinarian, academic, employment - with at least one being from a veterinarian

ENTRANCE REQUIREMENTS

Required undergraduate GPA: No minimum requirement

Mean GPA: for the 2016 matriculated class was 3.60 on a 4.00 scale

AP credits: must appear on official transcript

Course completion deadline: final grades/transcripts, including all required courses, must be received at CSU by July 15 prior to matriculation

Is a Bachelor's Degree Required? no

Is this an International School? no

ESTIMATED TUITION

Estimated Tuition Resident: $32,000

Estimated Tuition Contract: $32,000

Estimated Tuition Non-Resident: $58,000

AVAILABLE SEATS

Resident: 70

Non-resident: 30-35

Contract: 30-35

UAF/CSU: 10

TEST REQUIREMENTS

The GRE General Test (Verbal, Quantitative, Analytical) is required. The average GRE scores for the 2016 matriculated class are in the mid-150's for Verbal and Quantitative; and in the range of 4.0-4.5 for Analytical.

Test scores must be dated on or after August 1, 2012. It is the applicant's responsibility to schedule the test on or before August 11, 2017, so s/he can self-report unofficial scores on the Colorado Supplemental Application before the September 15, 2017, at 10:00 PM (MT) deadline. NOTE: The self-reported unofficial scores—Verbal, Quantitative, and Analytical—must be entered into the Colorado Supplemental Application in order to submit the application.

Sending official scores: Applicants should submit a request to their testing center, before September 15, to have official scores sent to CSU (code 4075; dept 0617—please use dept code). Official scores should be received at CSU by October 31. Official scores will be used to verify all applicant self-reported scores before offers are made.

VMCAS Participation: full

Accepts International Students? yes

ADDITIONAL INFORMATION

The veterinary program at CSU offers the following programs:

UAF (Alaska)/CSU: http://csu-cvmbs.colostate.edu/dvm-program/Pages/uaf-csu-collaborative-veterinary-program.aspx

MBA/DVM: http://csu-cvmbs.colostate.edu/dvm-program/Pages/DVM-MBA.aspx

MPH/DVM: http://csu-cvmbs.colostate.edu/dvm-program/Pages/DVM-MPH.aspx

MSA/DVM: http://csu-cvmbs.colostate.edu/dvm-program/Pages/dvm-msansci.aspx

MST/DVM: http://cs-cvmbs.colostate.edu/dvm-program/Pages/DVM-MST.aspx

PhD/DVM: http://csu-cvmbs.colostate.edu/dvm-program/Pages/DVM-PhD.aspx

FAVCIP (Food Animal): http://cs-cvmbs.colostate.edu/dvm-program/Pages/DVM-Special-Programs.aspx

http://csu-cvmbs.colostate.edu/dvm-program/Pages/DVM-Special-Programs.aspx

Application Deadline: 9/15/2017

PRE-VETERINARY PROFILE: CHRISTA CHEATHAM

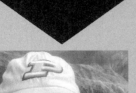

Current School Name
Purdue University

What type of veterinary medicine are you interested in pursuing, and why?
I am interested in either becoming an anatomic pathologist or a laboratory animal veterinarian. I am passionate about making discoveries in how human and animal health are related. I like to solve problems and I want to be an advocate for animals used in research.

What is/was your major during undergraduate school?
My major in undergraduate school was animal sciences.

What are your short-term and long-term goals?
My short-term goals are to be a successful veterinary student by learning the material and creating relationships with my professors. I also want to be involved with my community by teaching the public about the veterinary profession. My long-term goals would be to complete a residency to become board certified in pathology or laboratory animal so that I can teach and conduct research in academia.

What are you doing as an applicant/pre-vet to prepare for veterinary school?
To prepare for veterinary school, I have practiced good study habits and have taken high course loads every semester. I also have strived to get veterinary experience in a variety of areas such as small, large, and specialty sectors of veterinary medicine. I have been able to network with several veterinarians in the field I am interested in to be able to gain more experience.

What extracurricular activities are you involved in currently?
I am currently the fundraising chairman for Purdue's Pre-Veterinary Club. I am also the treasurer of the Heifer International Chapter. Both these clubs are interested in making the world a better place. I am involved in community service projects such as walking dogs for the Humane Society and serving meals to the homeless.

How old were you when you first became interested in being a veterinarian?
I was very young when I first became interested in becoming a veterinarian. I grew up on a beef cattle farm, so I frequently had to help the veterinarian give shots, do pregnancy checks, and pull calves during calving season.

Please describe your various experiences in preparation for applying to veterinary school.
I currently work as a veterinary assistant at a small animal clinic and as a research consultant for a mouse embryology laboratory. I've also worked in a histopathology laboratory, cared for laboratory animals, and have worked as a veterinary assistant in Purdue's oncology department. Additionally, I have conducted a few small research projects studying canine gait analysis and the impact that botulinum neurotoxin has on muscle contraction in mice.

What characteristics are you looking for in a veterinary school?
I am looking for a veterinary school that has a good comparative research program because it's what I am interested in. I look for faculty in pathology or lab animal medicine so that they could possibly be a mentor to me when I am a student. I also am looking for a school that has a lower tuition cost and is in an area where the cost of living is lower.

What advice do you have for other pre-veterinary students?
Never give up on your dreams. Make sure you get adequate experience in several areas of veterinary medicine to make sure that this is what you want to do. Have a plan to pay off your loans and prepare yourself for the stresses of being a veterinary student and veterinarian.

NEW YORK
CORNELL UNIVERSITY

Email Address: vet_admissions@cornell.edu
Website: http://www.vet.cornell.edu/admissions

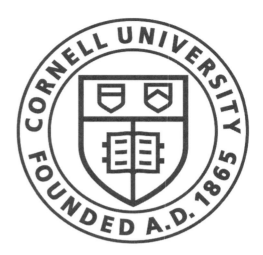

SCHOOL DESCRIPTION

Cornell is located in Ithaca, a college town of about 30,000 in the Finger Lakes region of upstate New York, a beautiful area of rolling hills, deep valleys, scenic gorges, and clear lakes. The university's 740-acre campus is bounded on two sides by gorges and waterfalls. Open countryside, state parks, and year-round opportunities for outdoor recreation, including excellent sailing, swimming, skiing, hiking, and other activities, are only minutes away.

> The curriculum is interdisciplinary and focuses on the student as the primary force in learning.

Ithaca is one hour by air and a four-hour drive from New York City, and other major metropolitan areas are easily accessible. Direct commercial flights connect Ithaca with New York, Boston, Chicago, Pittsburgh, Philadelphia, and other cities.

The tradition of academic excellence, the cultural vigor of a distinguished university, and the magnificent setting create a stimulating environment for graduate study. The curriculum differs from other programs in that it is interdisciplinary, small group learning early in the program and focuses on the student as the primary force in learning.

APPLICATION INFORMATION

For specific information about the application process visit our web site at: http://www.vet.cornell.edu /admissions

You may also subscribe to our free electronic Pre-Vet Newsletter at: http://www.vet.cornell.edu/admissions/PreVet Newsletters.cfm for application updates and current information about the College of Veterinary Medicine.

Residency implications: approximately 65 seats for New York State residents and 55 seats for non-NY residents

SUMMARY OF ADMISSION PROCEDURES

VMCAS application deadline: Friday, September 15, 2017 at 12 Midnight Eastern Time

Date acceptances emailed: January

Information sessions at the college for admitted students and alternates: February

School begins: mid/late August

Deposit (to hold place in class): $500.00 (by April 15, unless the 15th falls on a weekend, then the deposit deadline will be the following Monday)

Deferments: considered on an individual basis, and ordinarily granted for illness or other situations beyond the control of the applicant.

EVALUATION CRITERIA

The following admissions formula allows the applicant to see how their application will be reviewed:

25% Overall GPA

25% GRE (verbal & quantitative) or MCAT Scores

20% Animal/Veterinary/Biomedical Research Experiences

• at least one letter of evaluation from a veterinarian is required

PREREQUISITES FOR ADMISSION

Course Description	Number of Semester Credits	Necessity
English composition/writing-intensive courses (full year)	6	Required
Biology or zoology, full year with laboratory	6	Required
Physics, full year with laboratory	6	Required
Inorganic (or general) chemistry, full year with laboratory	6	Required
Organic chemistry, one semester	3	Required
Biochemistry, half year required; full year preferred	4	Required
Advanced Life Science course	3	Required
Non-prerequisite elective credits needed	26	Required

5% Quality of Academic Program

• with academic letter of evaluation

10% Non-Cognitive Skills

10% All Other Achievements

5% Personal Statement

ENTRANCE REQUIREMENTS

Required undergraduate GPA: No specific GPA requirement, but the grade range of those admitted tends to be 3.00-4.00.

AP credit policy: accepted for physics and general or inorganic chemistry with a score of 4 or higher.

Course completion deadline: all but 12 semester credits (or 18 quarter credits) of the prerequisite coursework should be completed at the time of application, with at least one semester of any two-semester series underway. Any outstanding prerequisites must be completed by the end of the spring term prior to matriculation.

Is a Bachelor's Degree Required? no

Is this an International School? no

ESTIMATED TUITION

Estimated Tuition Resident: $33,732

Estimated Tuition Contract: n/a

Estimated Tuition Non-Resident: $49,492

AVAILABLE SEATS

Resident: tentative 65

Contract: 0

Non-Resident: tentative 55

TEST REQUIREMENTS

Standardized examinations: Graduate Record Examination (GRE), general test (verbal and quantitative), or the Medical College Admission Test (MCAT) is required. Official test scores must be received directly from ETS or AAVMC by September 15. Test scores older than five years will not be accepted. TOEFL scores for international applicants whose first language is not English (and whose education was taught in a language other than English) should be received by this deadline as well.

VMCAS Participation: full

Accepts International Students? yes

ADDITIONAL INFORMATION

Combined Degree Programs

Combined DVM/PhD Program: By integrating Cornell's veterinary and graduate curricula in the DVM/PhD Program, we prepare students to become leaders in science, medicine, and society, able to excel in basic research, cutting-edge medicine, and teaching. Students receive substantial financial funding incentives to complete both degrees.

DVM/MPH (Masters in Public Health): A partnership between the College of Veterinary Medicine and the University Of Minnesota School Of Public Health allows students the opportunity to earn a Master of Public Health (MPH) degree while completing their DVM training.

For more information on both combined degree programs visit: http://www.vet.cornell.edu/admissions/OADualDegree.cfm

Other Admissions Programs

Sophomore Early Acceptance Program: The Early Acceptance Program gives exceptionally well qualified applicants the opportunity to obtain admission to veterinary school after the completion of the sophomore year and start the veterinary curriculum after completion of the junior year. With admission to the Cornell University College of Veterinary Medicine secured, the successful applicant may use the time between acceptance and matriculation to pursue experience in areas of personal interest. More information can be found at: https://www2.vet.cornell.edu/education/doctorveterinary-medicine/admissions/early-acceptance

Transfer Student Admissions: Cornell will consider applications for advanced standing in the DVM program on an individual basis, if an opening exists in the second-year class. More information can be found at: http://www.vet.cornell.edu/admissions/transfer_students.cfm

Summer Research Opportunities

The Leadership Program for Veterinary Scholars: A unique summer learning experience for veterinary students who seek to broadly influence the veterinary profession through a career in research. The program in an intensive research-oriented learning experience that combines faculty-guided research with career counseling, student-directed learning, and a variety of professional enrichment activities.

Additional Summer Research Opportunities: Additional summer research opportunities for veterinary students include the Veterinary Investigator Program, Veterinary Training in Biomedical Research, Aquavet, Summer Dairy Institute, the Food Animal Medicine Externship, and the Havemeyer Foundation Equine Research Fellowships.

For more information about all of these summer research opportunities visit: http://www.vet.cornell.edu/BBS/Scientists/SummerResearch.cfm

Other

Masters in Public Health at Cornell University: Beginning fall 2017 a campus-wide MPH program. Founded on the One Health paradigm. For more information: https://www2.vet.cornell.edu/education/graduate-studies/master-public-health-mph.

Application Deadline: VMCAS 9/15/2017

UNIVERSITY OF FLORIDA

Email Address: studentservices@vetmed.ufl.edu
Website: http://www.vetmed.ufl.edu

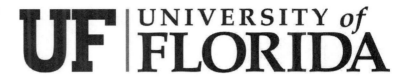

SCHOOL DESCRIPTION

The University of Florida is located in Gainesville, a college town of approximately 125,000 in north central Florida, midway between the Gulf of Mexico and the Atlantic Ocean. Changes in season are marked, but winters are mild and permit year-round participation in outdoor activities.

The university accommodates about 50,000+ students with programs in almost all disciplines. The College of Veterinary Medicine is a component of the Institute of Food and Agricultural Sciences (which also includes Agriculture and Forest Resources and Conservation). It is also one of 6 colleges affiliated with the Health Science Center (the other 5 are Dentistry, Public Health and Health Professions, Medicine, Nursing, and Pharmacy).

> The veterinary curriculum is a 9-semester program consisting of core curriculum and elective experiences.

The veterinary curriculum is a 9-semester program consisting of core curriculum and elective experiences. The core provides the body of knowledge and skills common to all veterinarians. The first four semesters concentrate primarily on basic medical sciences. In the first four semesters, students are also introduced to physical diagnosis, radiology, and clinical problems. They also spend time preparing for the clinical experience in a clinical techniques simulation laboratory and in the hospital by participating in supervised patient care. The core also includes experience in each of the specialized clinical areas and primary care. Elective areas of concentration permit students to investigate further the aspects of both basic and clinical sciences most relevant to their interests (e.g., small animal, food animal, equine, etc.). Students may also participate in optional Certificate Programs and/or the Joint DVM/MPH Program.

APPLICATION INFORMATION

For specific application information (availability, deadlines, fees, and VMCAS participation), please refer to the contact information listed above.

Residency implications: Florida has no contractual agreements. The college admits 88 Florida residents and 24 Non-Sponsored applicants each academic year. International applicants are included in the Non-Sponsored pool.

SUMMARY OF ADMISSION PROCEDURES

VMCAS application deadline: Friday, September 15, 2017 at 12 Midnight Eastern Time

UF Professional School Application deadline: Friday, September 15, 2017. Information on our supplemental requirements can be found at:

http://education.vetmed.ufl.edu/admissions/application

Date interviews are held: January/February

Date acceptances mailed: March

School begins: mid-August

Deposit (to hold place in class): none required

Deferments: considered on an individual basis

PREREQUISITES FOR ADMISSION		
Course Description	Number of Hours/Credits	Necessity
Biology (general, genetics, microbiology)	15	Required
Chemistry (inorganic, organic, biochemistry)	19	Required
Physics	8	Required
Mathematics (statistics)	3	Required
Humanities	9	Required
Social sciences	6	Required
English (2 courses in English composition)	6	Required
Electives	5	Required

EVALUATION CRITERIA

Academic Assessment

The University of Florida College of Veterinary Medicine (UFCVM) does not have a set minimum academic requirement in order to be admitted. However, Science, Last 45 and Overall GPAs in addition to GRE scores will be used in evaluating the academic ranking of applicants. Candidates are ranked in two independent applicant pools: Sponsored (Florida residents) and Non-Sponsored.

Full Application Review

Applicants selected from the academic ranking will have their entire vet school application reviewed individually by three members of the UFCVM Admissions Committee. Once again, there will be two applicant pools: Sponsored and Non-Sponsored, and the candidates will be scored and ranked on the following criteria:

Academic History and Experience: Academic load, number of withdrawals, research participation, teaching assistant positions, strength of academic references (if any), and academic flags/concerns.

Pre-Veterinary Experience and Preparation: Amount of legitimate pre-veterinary experience, amount of legitimate animal experience, strength of veterinary/animal-related references, relationship with references, and veterinary/animal experiences.

Overall Professionalism and Readiness to Matriculate: Overall professionalism of the application, strength of written communication skills, extracurricular experiences, community involvement, international experiences, awards and recognitions, non-veterinary or animal related employment experiences.

Candidate Interview

In early-to-mid February candidates selected from the full application review pool, will be invited to participate in the Interview process. Each applicant will be interviewed by a panel of two members of the Admissions Committee and one upper division Veterinary Student.

ENTRANCE REQUIREMENTS

Suggested undergraduate GPA: a minimum GPA of 3.00 on a 4.00 scale. The class of 2020 had an overall mean science prerequisite GPA of 3.58.

Course completion deadline: Applicants are expected to complete 80% of the Science and Math prerequisite courses before submitting an application.

Is a Bachelor's Degree Required? no

Is this an International School? no

ESTIMATED TUITION

Estimated Tuition Resident: $28,787

Estimated Tuition Contract: $0

Estimated Tuition Non-Resident: $45,500

AVAILABLE SEATS

Resident: 88

Contract: 0

Non-Resident: 24

TEST REQUIREMENTS

Standardized examinations: The Graduate Record Examination General Test is required. To be considered for Class of 2022 admissions cycle, the last day to sit for the GRE is August 31, 2017. We must have official GRE scores in our office by the September 15 deadline.

VMCAS Participation: full

Accepts International Students? on a case-by-case basis

ADDITIONAL INFORMATION

Supplemental Application Deadline: 9/15/2017

UNIVERSITY OF GEORGIA

Email Address: dvmadmit@uga.edu
Website: http://www.vet.uga.edu/admissions

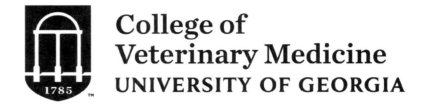

**College of
Veterinary Medicine**
UNIVERSITY OF GEORGIA

SCHOOL DESCRIPTION

The University of Georgia is located in Athens-Clarke County, with a population of over 100,000. Georgia's Classic City is a prospering community that reflects the charm of the Old South while growing in culture and industry (www. visitathensga.com). Athens is just over an hour away from the north Georgia mountains and the metropolitan area of Atlanta, and just over 5 hours away from the Atlantic coast.

> The University of Georgia has grown into an institution with 16 schools and colleges and more than 2,889 faculty.

In 1785, Georgia became the first state to grant a charter for a state-supported university. In 1801 the first students came to the newly formed frontier town of Athens. The University of Georgia has grown into an institution with 16 schools and colleges and more than 2,889 faculty members and 34,519 students.

APPLICATION INFORMATION

For specific application information (availability, deadlines, fees, and VMCAS participation), please refer to the contact information listed above.

Residency implications: Georgia retains up to 19 positions for contract students. Contracts are with Delaware (maximum 2 seats) and South Carolina (maximum 17 seats). The balance of those admitted are residents of Georgia or nonresident, non-contract applicants. International applications are accepted. Total number of students admitted each year: 114.

SUMMARY OF ADMISSION PROCEDURES

VMCAS application deadline: Friday, September 15, 2017 at 12 Midnight Eastern Time

Supplemental application deadline: September 15, 2017 at 1 PM Eastern Time (The deadline to request a supplemental application account will be posted on our website).

GRE score deadline: September 15, 2017 (scores must be submitted electronically from ETS) (Applicant must use code 5752).

Decision letters mailed: early–middle February

School begins: mid-August. A required 3-day orientation will precede the start of classes.

Deposit (to hold place in class): $500; $750 for non-resident, non-contract students.

Deferments: one-year deferments considered on a case-by-case basis.

EVALUATION CRITERIA

The admissions procedure includes a file evaluation. There are no interviews.

ADDITIONAL REQUIREMENTS AND CONSIDERATIONS

Program of Study
Animal/Veterinary Experience
References
Employment History
Personal Statement
Extracurricular Activities
Entrance Requirements

To view our prerequisite courses for admission to the UGA College of Veterinary Medicine please visit our website at vet.uga.edu/admissions/requirements.

Required undergraduate GPA: cumulative GPA of 3.00 or greater on a 4.00 scale or a combined score on the GRE verbal and quantitative sections of 1200 on the old scale or 308 or higher on the new scale.

Is a Bachelor's Degree Required? no

Is this an International School? no

ESTIMATED TUITION

Estimated Tuition Resident: approx. $19,010

Estimated Tuition Contract: approx. $19,010

Estimated Tuition Non-Resident: $47,380

AVAILABLE SEATS

Resident: 80

Contract: 17

Non-Resident: 17

TEST REQUIREMENTS

Standardized examinations: Graduate Record Examination (GRE) general test (including the analytical writing portion) must be completed within the 5 years immediately preceding the deadline for receipt.

VMCAS Participation: full

Accepts International Students? yes

ADDITIONAL INFORMATION

Combined DVM-graduate degree programs are available:

DVM-MPH Veterinarians in Public Health

DVM/PhD Veterinary Medical Scientist Training Program

Application Deadline: 9/15/2017

VMCAS Application Deadline: 9/15/2017

UNIVERSITY OF ILLINOIS

Email Address: admissions@vetmed.illinois.edu
Website: http://vetmed.illinois.edu

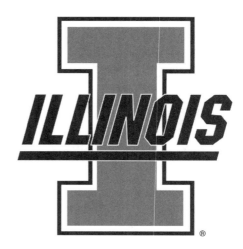

SCHOOL DESCRIPTION

The University of Illinois is in Urbana-Champaign, a community of 100,000 people located 140 miles south of Chicago. It is served by airports in Champaign, Chicago, Indianapolis, and St. Louis, 3 interstate highways, bus, and rail. The twin cities and university make a pleasant community with easy access to all areas and facilities. The university has 45,000 students and more than 11,000 faculty and staff members. It is known for its high-quality academic programs and its exceptional resources and facilities. It is the first university to have established a division of student disability resources. The university library has the largest collection of any public university and ranks third among all U.S. academic libraries. The university also has outstanding cultural and sports facilities and activities.

> It is known for its high-quality academic programs and its exceptional resources and facilities.

The College of Veterinary Medicine is located at the south edge of the campus. In addition to 500 students, the college has about 100 graduate students plus a full complement of residents and interns. There are more than 100 full-time faculty with research interests in a variety of biomedical sciences and clinical areas. This research activity offers a broad variety of experiences for students. The college also offers students a dynamic, integrated core-elective curriculum to prepare for careers in almost any area of the profession.

APPLICATION INFORMATION

For specific application information (availability, deadlines, fees, and VMCAS participation), please refer to our website: http://vetmed.illinois.edu/education/doctor-veterinary-medicine-degree/admissions

Supplemental questions specific to the University of Illinois are required and may be obtained from the Illinois page of the VMCAS application.

International applications are considered, although there are obvious constraints regarding translation of grades. The TOEFL will be required of any successful applicant before matriculation. U.S. Visa constraints may also be restrictive for admission.

Residency implications: priority is given to approximately 70 Illinois residents and 60 non-Illinois residents per class.

SUMMARY OF ADMISSION PROCEDURES

VMCAS application deadline: Friday, September 15, 2017 at 12 Midnight Eastern Time

Informational program and required interviews: mid-February

Date acceptances mailed: late February-early March

National application acceptance date: April 16, 2018

School begins: August 27, 2018

Deposit (to hold place in class): $500 deposit required on acceptance. Please check the Illinois Admissions website for the most current information.

Deferments: considered on an individual basis by the Associate Dean for Academic and Student Affairs.

EVALUATION CRITERIA

A 3-part admission procedure is used. An academic evaluation and an application evaluation of veterinary, animal experience and personal qualities are followed by a personal interview.

Academic evaluation: GRE test scores; Illinois science GPA; cumulative GPA; rigor of academic preparation

Nonacademic evaluation: veterinary-related experience, animal-related experience, community involvement, leadership, citizenship, and letters of recommendation; interview

ENTRANCE REQUIREMENTS

Required undergraduate GPA: a minimum cumulative GPA of 2.75 and a minimum Illinois science GPA of 2.75 on a 4.00 scale are required. The average statistics for students passing Admissions Phase I in 2014 were 3.59 cumulative GPA, 3.44 science GPA, and 65% GRE composite percentile

AP credit policy: AP credit is allowed to meet the 8 s.h. physics prerequisite requirement if a student is awarded the full 8 s.h. AP credit is allowed for biology and chemistry if it is followed up by more advanced college-level courses in those science areas.

GRE test within two years of application. Refer to website for specific dates.

Is a Bachelor's Degree Required? no

Is this an International School? no

ESTIMATED TUITION/FEES

Estimated Tuition Resident: $27,169 plus fees

Estimated Tuition Contract: not applicable

Estimated Tuition Non-Resident: $48,672 plus fees

AVAILABLE SEATS

Resident: 70

Contract: 0

Non-Resident: 60

TEST REQUIREMENTS

Standardized examinations: Graduate Record Examination (GRE), general test, is required. Test must be taken by September 1, 2017 for the 2017/2018 admission cycle. Test dates must be between August 1, 2015 and September 1, 2017. Tests outside this window will not be acceptable.

VMCAS Participation: full

Accepts International Students? yes

ADDITIONAL INFORMATION

Combined DVM/PhD programs may be available.

DVM/MPH with concurrent enrollment at University of Illinois at Chicago School of Public Health are also available.

Application Deadline: 9/15/2017

PRE-VETERINARY PROFILE: BRIANNA NAIZIR

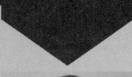

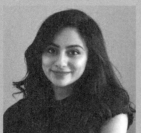

Current School Name
Macaulay Honors College at the City College of New York

What type of veterinary medicine are you interested in pursuing, and why?
Over the course of my career as an undergrad, I have always been interested in pursuing companion animal veterinary medicine. It has always been a dream of mine to be able to give back to my community and to have some sort of impact on communities around the world. Many neighborhoods in New York City do not have access to affordable veterinary care for their pets. I've also found that this issue is even more pressing in other places I've visited. After multiple trips to Puerto Rico to visit family, I realized just how alarming the number of stray and deathly ill dogs there were across the entire island. This issue is so prominent that Puerto Rico is sometimes called "dead dog island." As a small animal veterinarian, it will be my goal to provide veterinary care in communities that have little to no access to it.

Furthermore, many experiences I've had with animals outside of the traditional small-animal clinic have sparked my interest in other fields, such as exotic or zoo medicine. In addition to the fact that studying wildlife is absolutely fascinating, I feel that this field is becoming increasingly essential in our changing world. I would also like to contribute to wildlife conservation efforts by specializing in one of the relevant fields.

What is/was your major during undergraduate school?
As a current third-year undergraduate student, I am majoring in biology. The aspect of my major that I love the most is its versatility. I have been able to take classes in subjects that I had already had an interest in, such as ecology and evolution. I also have had the opportunity to explore and grow to love new biological topics. For instance, after taking a course in genetics, I fell in love with the field and decided to go forth and take epigenetics, as well as work in a lab that employs methods of genetics and microbiology.

What are your short-term and long-term goals?
Currently, my short term goal is to focus on my veterinary school application and to ultimately attend veterinary school. In addition to studying to take the GRE, I am constantly looking into new internships and extracurricular opportunities to gain exposure to the field.
My long-term goal is to become a companion animal veterinarian, specialize in exotics, and open up my own clinic. I would like to run a relatively small practice and also have a mobile clinic service. I will probably have my clinic in my native city of New York City and use my mobile clinic to travel to numerous low-income areas to provide free or low-cost veterinary care. This would include basic vaccinations, as well as spaying and neutering. Ultimately, my goal is to establish an animal sanctuary in upstate New York.

What are you doing as an applicant/pre-vet to prepare for veterinary school?
In order to prepare for veterinary school, I have founded a pre-veterinary society at my university. The objective of my club is to unite all students who share the same passion and to share resources needed to prepare for the vet school application process. Since the founding of my club, we have hosted speakers from establishments such as the Staten Island Zoo, Cornell University, and the Royal Veterinary College of London. In addition, I have also shadowed small animal veterinarians and have volunteered at clinics, a zoo, and biology laboratories. My main objective in preparation for veterinary school is to gain exposure to as many fields within the sphere of veterinary medicine as possible.

What advice do you have for other pre-veterinary students?
A major piece of advice that I have for other pre-veterinary students is to not be intimidated by obstacles. Something that first intimidated me was the fact that there are so few veterinary schools, which makes the application process very competitive. However, I believe that if you are truly passionate about the field, the best thing you can do is simply immerse yourself in it. Gain as much experience as possible and although it will initially be stressful and daunting, the work will later not even feel like work at all.

IOWA STATE UNIVERSITY

Email Address: cvmadmissions@iastate.edu
Website: www.vetmed.iastate.edu

IOWA STATE UNIVERSITY
College of Veterinary Medicine

SCHOOL DESCRIPTION

The Iowa State University College of Veterinary Medicine is located in the heart of one of the world's most intensive livestock-producing areas, which provides diverse food-animal clinical and diagnostic cases. A nearby metropolitan area and a regionally recognized referral veterinary hospital provide experience in companion-animal medicine and surgery. A strong basic science education during the first two years prepares veterinary students for a wide range of clinical experiences during the last two years. The College of Veterinary Medicine provides education in a wide variety of animal species and disciplines and allows fourth-year students to spend time with private practitioners, other colleges, research facilities, and in other educational experiences. Opportunities for research exist in the outstanding research programs in neurobiology, immunobiology, infectious diseases, and numerous other areas. The nearby National Animal Disease Center and the National Veterinary Services Laboratories provide additional research opportunities. The world's premier State Diagnostic Laboratory is part of the college and provides students with experience that is unmatched by any other veterinary college in the world. Graduates are highly sought after and can typically choose among multiple job offers. Career development and placement opportunities are also provided.

> Iowa State University graduates are highly sought after and can typically choose among five or six job offers.

APPLICATION INFORMATION

The most current application information (availability, deadlines, fees, VMCAS participation), may be found at: http://vetmed.iastate.edu/academics/prospective-students/admissions

Supplemental Application: A supplemental application is required. The supplemental becomes available in early May and the link can be found at: http://vetmed.iastate.edu/academics/prospective-students/admissions

Residency implications: priority is given to Iowa residents for approximately 60 positions. Iowa contracts on a year-to-year basis with North Dakota, South Dakota and Connecticut. Iowa also has a formal educational alliance with Nebraska. Remaining positions are available for residents of noncontract states or international students.

SUMMARY OF ADMISSIONS PROCEDURES

Application deadline: Friday, September 15, 2017 at 12 Midnight Eastern Time

Date acceptances mailed: approximately December 20

School begins: late August

Deposit (to hold place in class): $500.00

Deferments: considered on a case-by-case basis

EVALUATION CRITERIA

The admission procedure consists of a review of each candidate's application and qualifications:
1. Academic factors include grades, test scores, and courseload.

PREREQUISITES FOR ADMISSION		
Course Description	Number of Hours/Credits	Necessity
General chemistry (1 year series w/lab)	7	Required
Organic chemistry (1 year series w/lab)	7	Required
Biochemistry	3	Required
Biology (1 year series w/labs)	8	Required
Genetics (Upper level Mendelian and molecular)	3	Required
Mammalian anatomy and/or physiology	3	Required
Oral communication (interpersonal, group or public speaking)	3	Required
English composition	6	Required
Social Science/Humanities	8	Required
Physics (Physics 1 - first semester of a 2 semester series with mechanics)	4	Required
Electives	8	Required

2. Nonacademic factors include essays, experience, recommendations, and leadership and personal development activities.
3. Interviews are conducted.

ENTRANCE REQUIREMENTS

Required undergraduate GPA: the minimum GPA required is 2.50 on a 4.00 scale. The most recent entering class had a mean GPA of 3.55.

AP credit policy: must be documented by original scores submitted to the university, and must meet the university's minimum requirement in the appropriate subject area. CLEP (College-Level Examination Program) credits accepted only for the arts, humanities, and social sciences.

Course completion deadline: It is preferred that prerequisite science courses be completed by the end of the fall term the year the applicant applies, and these must be completed with a C (2.0) or better to fulfill the requirement. However, up to 2 prerequisite science courses may be taken the spring term prior to matriculation. All other prerequisites must be completed by the end of the spring term prior to matriculation with a C (2.0) or better. Pending courses may not be completed the summer prior to matriculation. Pass-not pass grades are not acceptable.

Is a Bachelor's Degree Required? no

Is this an International School? no

ESTIMATED TUITION

Estimated Tuition Resident: $22,176

Estimated Tuition Contract: Varies by contract

Estimated Tuition Non-Resident: $49,066

AVAILABLE SEATS

Resident (approximate): 60
Contract: 41
Non-Resident (approximate): 48

TEST REQUIREMENTS

Standardized examinations: Graduate Record Examination (GRE), general test, is required. Either the new Revised GRE or the previous GRE will be accepted, but the scores must either go directly from GRE to VMCAS or to Iowa State University College of Veterinary Medicine (code 6315). For the most current GRE submission information, please see the VMCAS instructions.

VMCAS Participation: full

Accepts International Students? yes

KANSAS STATE UNIVERSITY

Email Address: admit@vet.k-state.edu
Website: http://www.vet.k-state.edu

KANSAS STATE
U N I V E R S I T Y

SCHOOL DESCRIPTION

Kansas State University in Manhattan, Kansas, is located 125 miles west of Kansas City near Interstate 70. With a population of about 70,000 including KSU, Manhattan is in an area surrounded by many historical points of interest in a rich agricultural area of north central Kansas. Recreational activities abound in Manhattan and the surrounding area with fishing, boating, camping, and hunting among the favorites. Sporting events, theater, concerts, and excellent parks contribute to the many activities available. Kansans enjoy the four seasons, each of which brings its own special activities and events.

> The College of Veterinary Medicine is located on 80 acres just north of the main campus in 3 connected buildings.

Kansas State University is on a beautiful 664-acre campus. The College of Veterinary Medicine opened in 1905. It is located on 80 acres just north of the main campus in 3 connected buildings.

APPLICATION INFORMATION

For specific application information (availability, deadlines, fees, and VMCAS participation), please refer to the contact information listed above.

Supplemental Application: Available at http://www.vet.k-state.edu/admissions/apply/ between June 1 and September 15.

Contract tuition: resident tuition

Resident seats: approximately 45

Nonresident seats: approximately 62

Contract seats: 5 with North Dakota

Residency implications: to be eligible to be in the Kansas pool of applicants, the applicant must be a Kansas resident for tuition purposes at the time of application. International applicants are considered. Kansas has a contract for students from North Dakota.

SUMMARY OF ADMISSION PROCEDURES

Timetable

VMCAS application deadline: Friday, September 15, 2017 at 12 Midnight Eastern Time

Kansas State University supplemental application deadline: postmarked by Thursday, Sepmteber 15, 2017

Kansas residents: mid-December interviews scheduled

Nonresident: early January interviews scheduled

North Dakota: February interviews scheduled

Date acceptances mailed: within 6 weeks after interview

School begins: mid-August

Deposit (to hold place in class): $500.00

Deferments: may be considered by Admissions Committee for extraordinary circumstances.

EVALUATION CRITERIA

An admission procedure is used including evaluation of science grades, evaluation of all 3 GRE scores, assessment of the application and narrative, and a personal interview.

PREREQUISITES FOR ADMISSION

Course Description	Number of Hours/Credits	Necessity
Expository Writing I and II	6	Required
Public Speaking	2	Required
Chemistry I and II	8	Required
General Organic Chemistry w/lab	5	Required
General Biochemistry	3	Required
Physics I and II	8	Required
Principles of Biology or General Zoology	4	Required
Microbiology w/lab	4	Required
Genetics	3	Required
Social Sciences and/or Humanities	12	Required
Electives	9	Required

30%: Prerequisite science GPA

40%: Test scores

30%: Interview score including:

> References
>
> Animal/veterinary experience
>
> Leadership in college and community
>
> Autobiographical essay

ENTRANCE REQUIREMENTS

Prerequisites for Admission: Science courses must have been taken within six years of the date of enrollment in the professional program.

Required undergraduate GPA: the minimum required GPA to qualify for an interview is 2.80 on a 4.00 scale in both the prerequisite courses and the last 45 semester hours of undergraduate work. The most recent entering class had a mean prerequisite science GPA of 3.50.

AP credit policy: must appear on official college transcripts and be equivalent to the appropriate college-level coursework.

Course completion deadline: prerequisite courses must be completed by the end of the spring term of the year in which admission is sought.

Standardized examinations: Graduate Record Examination (GRE), general test, scores are required by September 15, unless all prerequisites are completed at Kansas State University.

ADDITIONAL REQUIREMENTS AND CONSIDERATIONS

Animal/veterinary work experience and knowledge

Employment record

3 evaluations required by nonfamily members: one veterinarian, one academic or preprofessional advisor, one professor or other professional.

Is a Bachelor's Degree Required? no

Is this an International School? no

ESTIMATED TUITION

Estimated Tuition Resident: $26,000

Estimated Tuition Contract: $26,000

Estimated Tuition Non-Resident: $56,000

AVAILABLE SEATS

Resident: 45

Contract: 5

Non-Resident: about 62

TEST REQUIREMENTS

Graduate Record Examination (GRE), general test

VMCAS Participation: full

Accepts International Students? yes

ADDITIONAL INFORMATION

Dual-Degree Programs

Combined DVM-graduate degree programs are available.

Combined DVM-MPH degree programs are available.

Early Admission Program

The Veterinary Scholars Early Admission Program is designed for those students having a genuine desire to enter the veterinary profession who attend Kansas State University with an ACT score of 29 or greater or an equivalent SAT score and who complete a successful interview during the fall semester of their freshman undergraduate year.

Application Deadline: 9/15/2017

LINCOLN MEMORIAL UNIVERSITY

Email Address: veterinaryadmissions@LMUnet.edu
Website: vetmed.lmunet.edu

LMU
Lincoln Memorial University

SCHOOL DESCRIPTION

Lincoln Memorial University (LMU) is an accredited, nonprofit university founded in 1897 through Abraham Lincoln's desire to provide an outstanding university for the people of Appalachia. The LMU main campus is located in Harrogate, Tennessee, beautifully situated at the foot of the historic Cumberland Gap and occupies more than 1,000 wooded acres with modern educational facilities that include classrooms and laboratories equipped with smart technology. Preclinical courses are taught at both the main Harrogate campus and at the DeBusk Veterinary Teaching Center (DVTC), utilizing state-of-the-art technology and clinical facilities about 15 minutes away from main campus in Ewing, Virginia.

> Hands-on animal and clinical skills-based experiences start in the first semester.

The goal of our innovative curriculum is to produce confident, practice-ready veterinarians by emphasizing clinical and professional skills. All students receive a well-rounded education in small animal medicine, bovine and equine medicine as well as exposure to avian and exotic animal medicine.

Features of the LMU-CVM program:

- Hands-on animal and clinical skills-based experiences start in the first semester and continuing throughout the entire curriculum.
- The large animal component of the DVTC provides a working farm environment with a large cattle and horse herd.
- Clinical Year Hybrid Distributive Education program prepares students by giving them the experience working in both primary care and specialty private practice environments. Students have the flexibility through clinical electives to focus on the facets of veterinary medicine that interest them the most such as food animal, research, or exotics.
- Veterinary research opportunities offer students valuable experience in this important facet of the profession. A diverse range of opportunities are available at LMU-CVM and with our partnership with the University of Kentucky.
- Case simulation labs teach professional and communication skills in an exam room environment with standardized patients in case scenarios.
- Students, staff, and faculty serve the health and wellness needs of people, animals, and the environment in Appalachia and beyond with an emphasis on the One Health approach.
- Our SOAR program provides small animal spays and neuters for the Appalachian region while providing valuable learning expertise for veterinary students.

Outside of classes, LMU-CVM students have the opportunity to participate in student clubs and activities. LMU is centrally located between Knoxville, TN, and Lexington, KY, two major cities that offer many cultural and recreational opportunities. The Cumberland Gap National Park is a favorite location for students to hike, run, bicycle, and relax between classes.

PREREQUISITES FOR ADMISSION		
Course Requirements	Semester Hours	Quarter hours
General Biology with lab	8	12
Genetics[1]	3	4
Biochemistry	3	4
Upper Division Science Electives (300 level or higher)[2]	8	12
Organic Chemistry with lab	6	9
General Chemistry with lab	8	12
Physics	3	4
English	6	9
Probability and Statistics	3	4
Social and Behavioral Sciences	6	9
Electives	6	9

[1] Animal breeding/reproduction courses must be approved by LMU-CVM
[2] Upper Division coursework (300 level or higher) including Anatomy, Cell Biology, Immunology, Microbiology, Molecular Biology, Physiology, Virology

APPLICATION INFORMATION

A complete application includes: VMCAS application, LMU-CVM supplemental application, and GRE scores. Late or incomplete applications will not be considered.

For more admissions details, please visit our website.

SUMMARY OF ADMISSIONS PROCEDURE

Timetable

Application materials due: Friday, September 15, 2017 at 12 Midnight Eastern Time

On-campus Interviews: September–February

Notification of decision: March

Deposit (to hold place in class): $1,250.00

Orientation/Classes Begin: early August

EVALUATION CRITERIA

Each completed application will receive a holistic review based on both academic and non-academic factors. Some considerations include:
- Overall GPA, Science GPA, GPA in last 2 years of study
- GRE Scores
- Leadership skills evidenced by participation in student and community organizations
- Well-rounded life experience that demonstrates a judicious balance of academic achievement, community service, and personal interests
- Experience in and knowledge of the veterinary profession
- Written communication skills as seen in a personal statement
- Letters of recommendation submitted via VMCAS

ENTRANCE REQUIREMENTS

Required undergraduate GPA: Applicants must have a cumulative GPA of at least 2.8 on a 4.00 scale. Students who don't meet the minimum GPA requirement, who have demonstrated a commitment to academic excellence (GPA > 3.2) in the last 2 years of study (45 semester hours) may be considered on a case-by-case basis.

Prerequisite completion: All prerequisite courses must be completed with grade of a C- or higher by the end of the Spring 2018 semester. All science prerequisites must have been completed in the last 10 years, or after August 2007.

AP credit policy: AP courses are accepted if they are specifically listed on an official college transcript and are equivalent to the appropriate college-level coursework.

Is a Bachelor's Degree Required? no

Is this an International School? yes

ESTIMATED TUITION

Tuition: $45,250 (subject to change)

As a nonprofit institution, tuition is the same for all LMU-CVM students, regardless of state residency.

AVAILABLE SEATS

Class size: 115

As a nonprofit institution, LMU does not have separate resident and nonresident seats.

TEST REQUIREMENTS

The Graduate Record Examination (GRE), general test, is required and scores are due by September 15. Exams taken prior to August 2014 will not be accepted. Applicants should schedule the GRE at least 30 days prior to the deadline.

Additional requirements: All applicants are required to complete the LMU-CVM Supplemental Application found on the LMU-CVM website.

VMCAS Participation: full

Accepts International Students? yes

ADDITIONAL INFORMATION

Application deadline: 9/15/2017

Further details about the application process and the LMU-CVM program can be found at: vetmed.lmunet.edu.

FOURTH-YEAR PROFILE: MEGAN MACNEILL

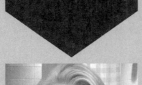
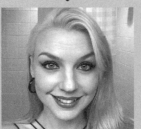

School you are attending
Murdoch University, Australia

What has been your favorite thing about attending veterinary school so far?
All of the different subjects learned and how different it is for each species. I also have enjoyed the tightknit group the veterinary class has become as you all have to work together to achieve goals and outcomes together. The teamwork and team building has been very enjoyable.

What advice do you have for prospective veterinary school applicants?
Keep an open mind and become friends with everyone you can at school. Their advice and friendship will help you immensely over the long run of your school and professional career.

What are your short-term / long-term goals?
My short-term goal is to commit more of what I am learning to memory. I have not been retaining information as well as I would like, so I am going to review and test myself more to commit important information to memory. My long-term goal is to help animals in need, such as shelter animals and injured or displaced wildlife.

What extracurricular activities are you involved in during veterinary school?
I take part in special-interest groups that attain speakers to come in and give us supplementary and specialised information about areas of veterinary interest such as business management, wildlife, or canines.

What was the biggest challenge you faced during veterinary school?
Time management—what projects and information should be studied when and for how long.

What advice do you have for other students who are currently in veterinary school?
It's all important information for the future. Try to retain the overall picture of your concepts as they will come into play for drug and disease management.

Why do you want to be a veterinarian?
To provide care for stray animals and to help conserve and protect wildlife and nature.

What field of veterinary medicine are you interested in pursuing and why?
Wildlife and shelter medicine. I wish to provide care to animals that are disadvantaged, displaced, or injured. I care very much about nature and conservation and wish to take part in conserving wild spaces and its inhabitants.

LOUISIANA STATE UNIVERSITY

Email Address: svmadmissions@lsu.edu
Website: www.lsu.edu/vetmed

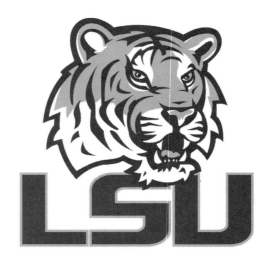

SCHOOL DESCRIPTION

The Louisiana State University campus is located in Baton Rouge, which has a population of more than 500,000 and is a major industrial city, a thriving port, and the state's capital. Since it is located on the Mississippi River, Baton Rouge was a target for domination by Spanish, French, and English settlers. The city bears the influence of all three cultures and offers a range of choices in everything from food to architectural design. Geographically, Baton Rouge is the center of south Louisiana's main cultural and recreational attractions. Equally distant from New Orleans and the fabled Cajun bayou country, there is an abundance of cultural and outdoor recreational activities. South Louisiana has a balmy climate that encourages lush vegetation and comfortable temperatures year round.

> Geographically, Baton Rouge is the center of south Louisiana's main cultural and recreational attractions.

The campus encompasses more than 2,000 acres in the southern part of Baton Rouge and is bordered on the west by the Mississippi River. The Veterinary Medicine Building, occupied in 1978, houses the academic departments, the veterinary library, the Louisiana Animal Disease Diagnostic Laboratory, the Wildlife Hospital of Louisiana, and the Veterinary Teaching Hospital. The school is fully accredited by the American Veterinary Medical Association.

APPLICATION INFORMATION

For specific application information (availability, deadlines, fees, and VMCAS participation), please refer to the LSU SVM admissions website at www.lsu.edu/vetmed/dvm_admissions.

Residency implications: The LSU SVM accepts 60-65 in-state residents and has approximately 9 seats reserved for AR contract students. The remaining 40-60 seats are offered to non-resident students. International students can be accepted as long as prerequisite courses have been taken in North America or coursework is certified as to U.S. equivalence.

SUMMARY OF ADMISSION PROCEDURES

Timetable

Suggested last date to take GRE: September 1

VMCAS application deadline: Friday, September 15, 2017 at 12 Midnight Eastern Time

Supplemental application deadline: All LSU SVM-specific questions in the VMCAS application must be completed as per the VMCAS instructions and by the VMCAS application deadline. (There is no supplemental application for the LSU SVM outside of the VMCAS application.)

LSU SVM application processing fee ($90) deadline: October 1

GRE score submission deadline: October 1

Date interviews are held: February*

Date acceptances mailed: early March

School begins: mid-August

*Interview invitations are extended to a select number of Louisiana, Arkansas, and out of state applicants as determined by the LSU SVM Admissions Committee.

PREREQUISITES FOR ADMISSION

Course Description	Number of Hours/Credits	Necessity
General Biology	8	Required
Microbiology (w/lab)	4	Required
Physics	6	Required
General Chemistry	8	Required
Organic chemistry	3	Required
Biochemistry	3	Required
English Composition	6	Required
Speech Communication	3	Required
Mathematics	5	Required
Electives	20	Required

Deposit (to hold place in class): $500.00 for non-residents only

Deferments: considered on a case-by-case basis

EVALUATION CRITERIA

The approximate components of the evaluation scoring are:

Objective evaluation:
GPA required courses: 29%
GPA last 45 hours: 18%
Test scores: 18%

Subjective evaluation:
Animal/veterinary experience, references: 15% (min. of 3 required, one by a veterinarian), essay, knowledge of profession, etc.
Personal interview: 10%
Committee evaluation: 10%

ENTRANCE REQUIREMENTS

Required undergraduate GPA: the minimum acceptable GPA for required coursework is 3.00 on a 4.00 scale. The mean GPA of the most recent entering class at the time of acceptance was 3.80.

AP credit policy: must appear on official college transcripts and be equivalent to the appropriate college-level coursework.

Is a Bachelor's Degree Required? no

Is this an International School? no

ESTIMATED ANNUAL TUITION

Estimated Tuition Resident: $26,828

Estimated Tuition Contract: $26,828

Estimated Tuition Non-Resident: $55,928

AVAILABLE SEATS

Resident: 60-65

Contract: 9

Non-Resident: 20-40

TEST REQUIREMENTS

Standardized examinations: The GRE revised General Test is required. The scores must be received no later than October 1. Note: All applicants must take the GRE revised General Test.

VMCAS Participation: full

Accepts International Students? The LSU SVM will accept international students as long as all prerequisite coursework has been completed at an accredited institution within the United States or Canada. Foreign coursework is not accepted in fulfillment of the course prerequisites.

ADDITIONAL INFORMATION

Application Deadline: 9/15/2017

MICHIGAN STATE UNIVERSITY

Email Address: admiss@cvm.msu.edu
Website: http://www.cvm.msu.edu

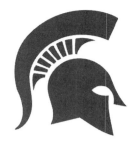

SCHOOL DESCRIPTION

Michigan State University's campus is bordered by the city of East Lansing, which offers sidewalk cafes, restaurants, shops, and convenient mass transit. The campus is traversed by the Red Cedar River and has many miles of bike paths and walkways. This park-like setting provides an ideal venue in which MSU's 48,906 students may enjoy outdoor concerts and plays, canoeing, and cross-country skiing. The campus is located in East Lansing, three miles east of Michigan's capitol in Lansing. It sits on a 5,200-acre campus with 2,100 acres in existing or planned development. There are 532 buildings which include 103 academic buildings.

> Michigan State University is a national leader in state-of-the-art technology and facilities.

TOP DISTINCTIONS

U.S. News & World Report ranks MSU 45th among the nation's public universities; 75% among the world's top 100 universities; first in the nation for 22 years for graduate programs in elementary; and secondary education. First in the nation for graduate programs in nuclear physics, organizational psychology, and rehabilitation counseling. One of the top 70 universities in the world.

The College of Veterinary Medicine is fortunate to have an outstanding faculty, all of whom hold the doctor of veterinary medicine degree and/or the doctor of philosophy degree. Nearly all of the specialty boards recognized by the American Veterinary Medical Association are represented on the faculty. Many of these faculty members are leaders in their fields, both nationally and internationally.

Today, the college includes four biomedical science departments—microbiology and molecular genetics, pathobiology and diagnostic investigation, pharmacology and toxicology, and physiology; two clinical departments—large-animal clinical sciences and small-animal clinical sciences; two service units—the Veterinary Medical Center and the Diagnostic Center for Population and Animal Health; and several research centers.

Michigan State has a long-standing commitment to equal opportunity, affirmative action, and multiculturalism. The College of Veterinary Medicine has attained national recognition for its leadership in programs for the encouragement of underrepresented groups at the preprofessional, professional, and advanced studies levels, as well as for increased diversity in its faculty.

APPLICATION INFORMATION

For specific application information (pre-requisite science courses, deadlines, and VMCAS participation), please refer to our website: http://cvm.msu.edu

Residency implications: priority is given to Michigan residents. Up to 37 positions are filled with nonresident and international applicants.

SUMMARY OF ADMISSION PROCEDURES

VMCAS application deadline: Friday, September 15, 2017 at 12 Midnight Eastern Time

Electronic evaluations to VMCAS: Friday, September 15, 2017 at 12 Midnight Eastern Time.

PREREQUISITES FOR ADMISSION

Course Description	Number of Hours/Credits	Necessity
English Composition	3	Required
Social and Behavioral Sciences	6	Required
Humanities	6	Required
General Inorganic Chemistry (with Laboratory)	3	Required
Organic Chemistry (with laboratory)	6	Required
Biochemistry (upper division)	3	Required
General Biology (with laboratory)	6	Required
College Algebra and Trigonometry	3	Required
College Physics (with laboratory)	8	Required
Advanced Biology Elective Course	3	Required

For the most accurate information about the prerequisites, please contact the Office of Admissions at admiss@cvm.msu.edu

Submit transcripts from *all* colleges attended to VMCAS by September 15, *including* colleges where you took courses that transfer to your main institution.

International transcripts must be evaluated by World Education Services (WES) and submitted to VMCAS. It is recommended that transcript(s) be submitted to the translation service at least one month prior to the deadline of September 15.

Non-refundable deposit (to hold place in class): (non-refundable) $500.00 for residents; $1,000.00 for non-residents

Deferments are rare.

ENTRANCE REQUIREMENTS

Required undergraduate GPA: The minimum required GPA for science prerequisite courses is 3.0 and for the last three semesters GPA is 3.0. The means for the most recent entering class were a science prerequisite GPA of 3.59 and a last three semester GPA of 3.77. The last three semester GPA includes a minimum of 36 credits for undergraduate students and a minimum of 18 credits for a graduate student.

AP credit policy: AP credit(s) must appear on an official transcript and be equivalent to appropriate college-level coursework.

Is a Bachelor's Degree Required? no

Is this an International School? no

ESTIMATED TUITION

Estimated Tuition Resident: $28,804

Estimated Tuition Contract: $0

Estimated Tuition Non-Resident: $56,546

AVAILABLE SEATS

Resident: 78

Contract: 0

Non-Resident: 37

TEST REQUIREMENTS

Standardized examinations: The GRE is not required. International applicants who are non-native speakers of English and who do not hold a bachelor's degree from a US institution must take a test of English as a second language. Options are the TOEFL iBT, the IELTS, or the CAEL.

VMCAS Participation: full

Accepts International Students? yes

ADDITIONAL REQUIREMENTS AND CONSIDERATIONS

Evaluation of written application (including veterinary/research experience)

Letters of recommendation (3 submitted by September 15, 2017, at 12 Midnight Eastern Time through VMCAS; 1 must be completed by a veterinarian)

Multiple Mini Interview or MMI

Acceptance deadline is Monday, April 16, 2018

2015-2016 ADMISSIONS SUMMARY

Number of Applicants: 955

Number of New Entrants

Resident: 78

Non-Resident/International: 37

Total: 115

EXPENSES AND FEES

Resident: $28,804

Non-resident: $56,546

EARLY ADMISSION PROGRAM

The Veterinary Scholars Admission Program has been established by the College of Veterinary Medicine in cooperation with the Honors College at Michigan State University. This program provides admission opportunity for students who wish to enter the four year professional veterinary medicine degree program after earning a bachelor's degree. The bachelor's degree program must include advanced and enriched coursework representing scholarly interest and achivements. Enrollment at MSU and membership in the Honors College are required to be eligible for this option. For information on Honors College membership, contact: Honors College, 105 Eustace-Hall, 468 E. Circle Drive, Michigan State University, East Lansing, MI 48824; telephone (517) 355-2326; or visit their website at http://honorscollege.msu.edu.

PRODUCTION MEDICINE PATHWAY

The Production Medicine Scholars Pathway has been established by the College of Veterinary Medicine in cooperation with the department of Animal Sciences at Michigan State University. This pathway is available to MSU Animal Science students who complete, in addition to the minimum pre-veterinary medicine requirements, a bachelor's degree in Animal Sciences with a concentration in production animal medicine. The concentration is designed to prepare students for a career in herd based, agricultural veterinary practice. The pathway provides an early admission option for Michigan State University students planing to earn a baccalaureate degree in Animal Science with a concentration in production medicine. Successful applicants must have a strong academic and non-academic credentials, a demonstrated interest in food animal production medicine and agricultural veterinary medicine. Additional information about the pathway may be obtained from 1250 Anthony Hall, 474 S. Shaw Lane, Department of Animal Science, Michigan State University, East Lansing, MI 48824 or visit the website: http://www.ans.msu.edu.

DUAL DEGREE PROGRAMS

Combined DVM-MPH degree program available

Combined online DVM/MS in Food Safety available

Application Deadline: 9/15/2017, midnight EST

MIDWESTERN UNIVERSITY

Email Address: admissaz@midwestern.edu
Website: http://www.midwestern.edu

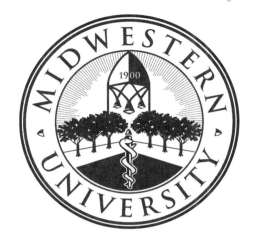

SCHOOL DESCRIPTION

The Midwestern University College of Veterinary Medicine (MWU-CVM) presents to its students a four year program leading to the Doctor of Veterinary Medicine (DVM) degree. The first 8 quarters are a mix of classroom lectures, laboratories, simulation lab exercises with virtual clients and patients, and small group, student-centered learning experiences. Hands-on live animal contact begins in the first quarter and continues throughout the program. Quarters 9-13 involve diverse clinical training, both on campus (about 85%) and at external sites (about 15%). Three new buildings, including a 111,000 square foot small animal Veterinary Teaching Hospital and a roughly 36,000 square foot large animal/pathology facility, insure our students will begin their careers in state-of-the-art surroundings.

> Three new buildings insure MWU-CVM students will begin their careers in state-of-the-art surroundings.

In October, 2014, the American Veterinary Medical Association Council on Education (AVMA-COE) extended provisional accreditation to the College. This notification indicates that the University and College submitted a plan which successfully met the 11 standards required by the AVMA to become accredited. The program will be eligible for full accreditation in 2018, upon graduation of the first class.

APPLICATION INFORMATION

The CVM utilizes the Veterinary Medical College Application Service (VMCAS). The VMCAS application is available online at www.aavmc.org. The VMCAS application cycle opens in June of each year. The official VMCAS application deadline is September 15, 2017 at 12 Midnight Eastern Time. Midwestern accepts direct applications after the close of the VMCAS cycle. Requests for withdrawing an application must be submitted in writing. In accordance with the Association of American Veterinary Medical Colleges acceptance deadline policy, students are not required to accept or reject an offer of admission until April 15. Students may accept or reject earlier if so inclined. If a signed letter accepting admission and the required deposit are not received by April 15, the offer of admission may be withdrawn.

SUMMARY OF ADMISSION PROCEDURES

Students seeking admission to the CVM must submit the following documented evidence:

1. Completion of prerequisite coursework or plans to complete the coursework prior to matriculation. (Confirmed by official transcripts)
    a. Minimum science AND minimum total cumulative GPA of 2.75 on a 4.00 scale.
    b. No grade lower than a C in any course will be accepted for credit. (Pass/fail and satisfactory/ unsatisfactory grading is not acceptable in prerequisite science courses.)
2. Completion of a minimum of 240 hours (6 weeks) of veterinary, health sciences, animal or biomedical

PREREQUISITES FOR ADMISSION		
Course Description	Number of Hours/Credits	Necessity
Biology	8	Required
Biochemistry	3	Required
Organic Chemistry with Lab	8	Required
Mathematics	6	Required
Physics with Lab	4	Required
English Composition	6	Required
Science Electives	8	Required

research experience. Students with additional hours of work experience will present a stronger case for admission.

3. Competitive scores on the GRE General Test.
4. Three letters of recommendation. (Students may submit up to 4 letters of recommendation.)
   a. At least one of the letters must be from a veterinarian.
   b. The other letters can be from other veterinarians, or from pre-veterinary or science professors, or from someone who can testify to the integrity and ethical standards of the applicant.
   c. Letters written by family members are not acceptable.
   d. Letters must be submitted by evaluators. Letters submitted by students are not accepted by the Office of Admissions.
5. Although not required, a Bachelor's degree will make a candidate more competitive.

ENTRANCE REQUIREMENTS

1. Demonstrate an understanding of the veterinary medical profession.
2. Demonstrate service orientation through community service or extracurricular activities.
3. Have a proper motivation for and commitment to the veterinary profession as demonstrated by previous salaried work, volunteer work, or other life experiences.
4. Possess the oral and written communication skills necessary to interact with patients, clients, and colleagues.

5. Pass the Midwestern University criminal background check.
6. Abide by Midwestern University's Drug-Free Workplace and Substance Abuse Policy.
7. Meet the Technical Standards for the College (see below).

Is a Bachelor's Degree Required? no

Is this an International School? no

ESTIMATED TUITION

Estimated Tuition Resident: $59,500

Estimated Tuition Contract: $59,500

Estimated Tuition Non-Resident: $59,500

AVAILABLE SEATS

100

TEST REQUIREMENTS

VMCAS Participation: full

Accepts International Students? yes

ADDITIONAL INFORMATION

Science electives include cell biology, physiology, microbiology, genetics, animal nutrition, etc.

Minimum of 64 total semester hours/96 quarter hours

Application Deadline: 9/15/2017

UNIVERSITY OF MINNESOTA

Email Address: dvminfo@umn.edu
Website: z.umn.edu/prospective

UNIVERSITY OF MINNESOTA

College of Veterinary Medicine

SCHOOL DESCRIPTION

The University of Minnesota College of Veterinary Medicine prepares future leaders in companion animal, food animal, and public health practice, as well as research and education. University of Minnesota students benefit from one of the largest teaching hospitals in the country, as well as world renowned faculty in zoonotic diseases, comparative medicine, and population systems. The College offers state-of-the-art facilities, including the Veterinary Medical Center, Leatherdale Equine Center, and the Raptor Center, which in 1988 became the world's first facility designed specifically for birds of prey. Off-site facilities include farms throughout Minnesota and around the world.

> Students gain hands-on experience throughout the entire program in clinical and professional skills courses.

The College of Veterinary Medicine is located on the 540-acre St. Paul campus. Students enjoy a small, intimate campus atmosphere of approximately 3,000 students while benefiting from the numerous amenities available within one of the nation's largest university systems.

The Twin Cities of Minneapolis and St. Paul have a combined population of approximately 2.5 million people and represents one of the largest metropolitan areas where a veterinary college is located. The Twin Cities is the cultural center for the region, abundant with outdoor recreational opportunities, and is repeatedly cited as one of the most livable metropolitan areas in the nation.

In 2013-14, the DVM program underwent a complete curriculum revision. During the first three years of the DVM program, students focus on the study of the normal animal, the pathogenesis of diseases and the prevention, alleviation and clinical therapy of diseases. Students gain hands-on experience throughout the entire program in clinical and professional skills courses.

The program concludes with thirteen months of clinical rotations in the Veterinary Medical Center, during which time students learn methods of veterinary care and develop skills needed for professional practice. Students can choose from over 65 rotations. The fourth year includes up to twelve weeks of externship experiences at off-campus sites of the student's choice.

APPLICATION INFORMATION

Application requirements include a complete VMCAS application, three electronic letters of reference submitted through VMCAS, official transcripts submitted through VMCAS, GRE examination scores, and an $85 application processing fee. The University of Minnesota College of Veterinary Medicine does not utilize a supplemental application.

The application, transcripts, and references are due to VMCAS by their respective deadlines.

All other application materials are due to the College by the application deadline of September 15, 2017 at 12 Midnight Eastern Time. For more application information, please visit z.umn.edu/prospective.

Residency implications: first priority is given to residents of Minnesota and residents of states with which a reciprocity or contract agreement exists (North Dakota and South Dakota). Residents of other states are encouraged to apply. International applicants should contact

PREREQUISITES FOR ADMISSION	
Course Description	**Number of Hours/Credits**
English (2 courses)	6
Algebra, Pre-Calculus, or Calculus	3
General Chemistry w/ Labs (2 courses, plus 2 labs)	6
Organic Chemistry	3
Bichemistry	3
General Biology w/ Lab	3
Zoology w/ Lab	3
Genetics	3
Microbiology w/ Lab	3
Physics (2 courses)	6
Liberal Education (3 courses)	9
Statistics	3

the Admissions Office for additional information. The University of Minnesota will accept 104 students into the program each year. Approximately 52 of the 104 seats are reserved for resident/reciprocity eligible applicants. Approximately 52 seats are held for non-resident applicants.

SUMMARY OF ADMISSION PROCEDURES

Timetable

VMCAS application deadline: Friday, September 15, 2017 at 12 Midnight Eastern Time

Date acceptances mailed: mid-February

School begins: last week of August

Deposit (to hold place in class): $500.00

Deferments: can be requested for extenuating circumstances that warrant a 1-year delay in admission. Requests to defer submitted after July 15 will not be considered.

EVALUATION CRITERIA

Objective measures of educational background

• GPA in prerequisite coursework

• GPA in most recent 45-semester credits

• GRE Test scores

Behavioral interviews

Subjective measures of personal experience

• Employment record

• Extracurricular and/or community service activities

• Leadership abilities

• References

• Maturity/reliability

• Animal/veterinary knowledge, experience, and interest

2016-2017 ADMISSIONS SUMMARY

Number of Number of Applicants / New Entrants

Resident: 156/52 admitted

Non-Resident: 655/52 admitted

Total: 811/104 admitted

The figures for new entrants include students taking delayed admission from the previous year.

*Includes residents of North and South Dakota

EXPENSES FOR THE 2016-2017 ACADEMIC YEAR

Tuition and fees

Residents: $31,420*

Nonresidents: $56,478*

*This includes all tuition and fees.

Students from Minnesota and South Dakota pay resident tuition rates. Students from North Dakota can apply to the state of North Dakota for tuition support through the Professional Student Exchange Program (PSEP). Approved North Dakota students pay resident tuition rates. North Dakota students not approved pay non-resident tuition rates. Students from all other states or international locations pay non-resident tuition rates.

Students may apply for residency after one year of enrollment.

ENTRANCE REQUIREMENTS

All prerequisites must be graded at a C- or better. Math and science prerequisites courses must be recent within ten years of the application deadline.

Liberal education requirements: A minimum of three courses (9 credits) designated as liberal education by the applicant's undergraduate institution attended.

Required undergraduate GPA: 2.75 minimum GPA required for prerequisite GPA and last-45 semester credit GPA. The class of 2020 had a mean GPA of 3.65 (on a 4.00 scale) for required courses and 3.73 for the last 60 quarter-hour or 45 semester-hour credits of coursework prior to admission.

AP credit policy: must appear on official college transcripts and be equivalent to the appropriate college-level coursework.

Course completion deadline: prerequisite courses must be completed by the end of the spring term (not later than June 15) of the academic year in which application is made. No more than five prerequisite science and math courses may be pending completion during the fall and spring semesters of the application cycle. Science laboratory courses are not included in the count of five.

Standardized examinations: Graduate Record Examination (GRE), general test, is required. Results must be received by the College by the application deadline. The mean combined score for the verbal and quantitative sections of the GRE for the class of 2020 was 312. When scheduling your exam, confirm your test date will allow enough time for results to be delivered by the application deadline. Send test results to institution code 6904.

Is a Bachelor's Degree Required? no

Is this an International School? no

ESTIMATED TUITION

Estimated Tuition Resident: $31,420

Estimated Tuition Contract: n/a

Estimated Tuition Non-Resident: $56,478

AVAILABLE SEATS

Resident: 52

Contract: n/a

Non-Resident: 52

TEST REQUIREMENTS

Graduate Record Exam

VMCAS Participation: full

Accepts International Students? yes

ADDITIONAL INFORMATION

Application Deadline: 9/15/2017

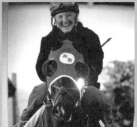

Current School Name
Virginia-Maryland Regional College of Veterinary Medicine (Virginia-Tech)

Why do you want to be a veterinarian?
My desire to be a veterinarian is probably the same as everyone else's: I like animals—horses in particular—and want to help them lead healthy lives. My sister and I were the neighborhood kids who fixed up lizards and baby birds! Since then, I have spent my life working with horses and can't imagine doing anything else. Now I have the opportunity to become a vet, so it will be great to combine the "helping" and "caring for" impulses with horses.

What are your short-term and long-term goals?
My short-term goals are to complete a six-week horse shoeing course this summer, and to complete one externship at a large-volume equine facility.

What did you do as an applicant to prepare for applying to veterinary school?
I came to vet school in a roundabout way, so I knew I needed to make sure all my academics were in order. As a non-traditional student (i.e., old!), I had completed my undergraduate science classes years ago, so I re-took some and added some more current classes. I also knew I had a lot of experience working with large animals, so I became a vet tech in a small animal clinic. This was very helpful, since I learned a lot of skills and had some great opportunities to learn about small animal disease and treatment.

What advice would you give to applicants or those considering applying to veterinary school?
My advice to current or potential applicants to veterinary school would be to work in the field you are considering. There are two benefits: you will gain experience, and you will also be able to save some money. I don't recommend "shadowing," since you only see one end of the job. If you want to go equine, for example, work as a groom. Whatever field you want to go into, find a job where you have to do the "hard yards" and see if you still love it.

What helped make the transition to veterinary school easier for you?
I have the most awesome friends in the world, and they reached out to me to make sure I was doing all right. They even sent care packages with cookies during exams! You will need a support system, since vet school is pretty grueling.

What is your advice on student debt?
I would suggest working to pay off all of your undergraduate debt before you apply to veterinary school. I know it seems like you will be losing too much time, but it will help financially, and it will give you more experience that will in the long run make you a better vet.

What are you most excited about learning in veterinary school?
Everything equine!

MISSISSIPPI STATE UNIVERSITY

Email Address: MSU-CVMAdmissions@cvm.msstate.edu

Website: http://www.cvm.msstate.edu

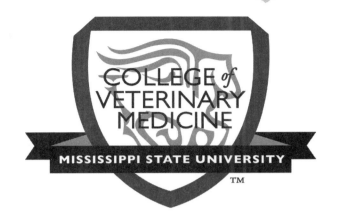

SCHOOL DESCRIPTION

Starkville is home to more than 21,000 MSU students and their Bulldogs. Starkville is located in northeast central Mississippi and has a population of 24,000. Being a land-grant university, MSU is green and beautifully landscaped. The university includes 9 farms scattered throughout the state. The College of Veterinary Medicine (the Wise Center) was completed in 1982. The college includes 620 rooms on 8 acres, or 360,000 square feet, under one roof.

The curriculum of the MSU-CVM is divided into 2 phases: Phase 1 or Pre-clinical (freshman and sophomore years) and Phase 2 or Clinical (junior and senior years).

Year 1 uses foundation courses to expose the student to important medical concepts and address multidisciplinary problems.

Year 2 is devoted to the study of clinical diseases and abnormalities of animal species. Surgery labs begin in the second year.

Year 3 is comprised of clinical rotations in the College's Animal Health Center, and elective courses.

Year 4 includes core rotations in internal medicine and ICU, large animal ambulatory, neurology, ophthalmology, and the Jackson Emergency/Referral Clinic.

The remainder of the fourth year is largely experiential and offers the student the opportunity to select among approved experiences in advanced clinical rotations, elective courses, and/or externships. The first 3 years of the curriculum are 9-10 months in length, while the fourth year is 12 months.

> The curriculum of the MSU-CVM is divided into 2 phases: Phase 1 or Pre-clinical and Phase 2 or Clinical.

APPLICATION INFORMATION

For specific application information (availability, deadlines, fees, and VMCAS participation), please refer to the contact information listed above.

Residency implications: Mississippi State accepts 40 Mississippi residents, 5 contract students from South Carolina, 7 contract students from West Virginia, and 40 non-resident applicants.

SUMMARY OF ADMISSION PROCEDURES

Timetable

VMCAS application deadline: Friday, September 15, 2017 at 12 Midnight Eastern Time

GRE General Exam scores and supplemental application deadline: September 15, 2017 at 12 Midnight Eastern Time. MSU will use September 15, 2017 as the date for supplemental applications.

Date interviews are held: January/February

Date acceptances mailed: February

First-year classes begin: early July

Deposit (to hold place in class): $500.00

Deferments: requests are considered on an individual basis

65

PREREQUISITES FOR ADMISSION		
Course Description	Number of Hours/Credits	Necessity
English Composition and/or Academic Writing	6	Required
Speech or Technical Writing	3	Required
Mathematics (College Algebra or higher)	6	Required
General Biology and accompanying labs	8*	Required
Microbiology with laboratory	4	Required
General Chemistry and accompanying labs	8*	Required
Organic Chemistry and accompanying labs	8*	Required
Biochemistry	3	Required
Physics (may be Trig-based)	6	Required
Advanced (upper-level) science electives	12	Required
Humanities, fine arts, social sciences and behavioral electives	15	Required

* indicates requirement of a minimum 6 hours of lecture and 2 hours of laboratory

EVALUATION CRITERIA

Grades (minimum competitive GPAs are typically 3.3-3.4)

Quality of academic program

Test scores

Animal/veterinary experience

Participation in extra-curricular and community service activities and outside employment

Leadership and interpersonal skills

References (3 required; one must be from a veterinarian)

Personal statement

Interview of applicants selected on basis of academic and non-academic criteria.

ENTRANCE REQUIREMENTS

Required undergraduate GPA: a minimum overall GPA of 2.8 on a 4.0 scale. The minimum GPA must be maintained throughout the application process. The class of 2020 has an average undergraduate GPA of 3.62.

No grade lower than a C- is acceptable in any required course throughout the application process (application through matriculation). Remediated and repeated courses must be completed before the application is submitted.

AP credit policy: must appear on official college transcripts and be equivalent to the appropriate college-level coursework.

Is a Bachelor's Degree Required? no

Is this an International School? no

2016-2017 TUITION AND FEES

Estimated Tuition Resident: $23,200

Estimated Tuition Contract: $23,200

Estimated Tuition Non-Resident: $46,400

AVAILABLE SEATS

Resident: 40

Contract: 12

Non-Resident: 40

TEST REQUIREMENTS

Standardized examinations: Graduate Record Exam (GRE), general test, is required (no minimum score) and is due at the school by September 15.

GRE must have been taken within 3 years of application deadline.

Students should schedule the GRE exam 30 days prior to deadline.

VMCAS Participation: full

Accepts International Students? yes

ADDITIONAL INFORMATION

DVM-PhD Program
The mission of the MSU-CVM DVM-PhD program is to prepare exceptional students for careers as veterinary scientists to meet the nation's critical needs in animal and human health research. It is the intent of the MSU-CVM DVM-PhD program to provide the full rigor of training from the DVM and PhD degrees as if they were pursued separately. The program is designed to integrate the research and clinical training programs so that students will experience a logical progression and level of responsibility throughout the program. It is also the intent of the program to provide a system of moral and financial support for the students who have committed to it.

APPLICATION PROCESS

The simultaneous pursuit of DVM and PhD degrees requires a highly motivated student who can handle a rigorous course load. Students seeking admission to this program go through a two-step interview process. The student is interviewed for admission into the DVM professional education program and the graduate program of the college. A student admitted to the DVM-PhD program takes graduate coursework and after two years begins the DVM professional education curriculum. Completion of the DVM-PhD program will require 7 years in most cases; however, this is 1 to 2 years shorter than the time required to complete both degrees if they were pursued separately.

PROGRAM STRUCTURE

An applicant granted admission to the DVM-PhD program will initiate his/her PhD coursework in the upcoming summer or fall semester and will remain engaged in graduate work until the fall semester two years later. Students admitted to the DVM-PhD program will have a position reserved in the DVM program two years subsequent to starting the DVM-PhD program as long as the student progressed appropriately during the initial two years of the PhD program. Upon successful completion of graduate coursework (maintaining a 3.0 GPA), a successful preliminary defense, and acceptance of a research proposal in the format of a federal agency grant proposal by the student's PhD committee, the student will continue in the DVM-PhD program and begin the DVM professional curriculum. Once the student has entered the DVM curriculum, he or she will matriculate through the DVM program with the same class he/she enters the curriculum with. The final year of the program will be spent completing the PhD research, writing, and defending the dissertation.

MSU-CVM EARLY ENTRY PROGRAM

The Early Entry Program is a unique program of the College of Veterinary Medicine (CVM) that allows high-achieving high school seniors to earn pre-acceptance (early, pre-approved acceptance) into the CVM.

Students who have an interest in veterinary medicine and meet application requirements during high school may apply for the Early Entry Program. If a student is accepted into this program, he/she begins undergraduate work at MSU after high school graduation, and completes the first three to four years of prerequisite courses, while also working toward completion of a bachelor's degree. After the student has completed all course requirements for the College of Veterinary Medicine, has remained in good standing, and has taken the GRE General Exam, he/she matriculates into the CVM as a pre-accepted student. The student does not make further application to the CVM.

Students applying for this program must have the following qualifications:
1. ACT composite score of 27 (SAT score of 1820 on new SAT); and
2. High school grade average of 90 (3.6 on a 4.0 scale)

In addition, the Early Entry Program Admissions Committee considers animal and veterinary experience, work experience, leadership qualities, and nontechnical skills and aptitudes (character, community service, etc.) as described in the applicant's written application to the Early Entry Program, and in the applicant's Letters of Recommendation (provided in the application).

Twenty-five positions are available each year. We normally receive 70 to 80 applications. Both Mississippi and out-of-state students are eligible for the program.

Applications for the Early Entry Program are available by October 1 each year, and are due for return by January 5. Applicants are notified of acceptance status by early February.

Applications are available online from October 1 through December 31. Please see the following website for the application and important information: http://www.cvm.msstate.edu/academics/early_entry_program.html

Application Deadline: 9/15/2017

UNIVERSITY OF MISSOURI

Email Address: seayk@missouri.edu
Website: http://cvm.missouri.edu/prospective.htm

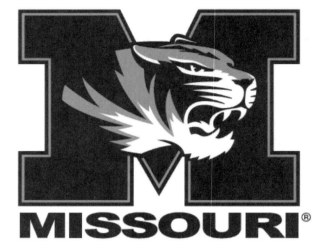

SCHOOL DESCRIPTION

The University of Missouri is located among rolling forested hills north of the famous Lake of the Ozarks. Columbia is noted for its high quality of life and low cost of living and is consistently rated among the best cities to live in by Money Magazine. The city abounds with walking trails, 3,000 acres of state park lands, federal forests, and wildlife refuges. Columbia is located between Kansas City and St. Louis-cities that have major-league sports teams and other big-city recreational amenities. Columbia itself offers SEC Conference football, basketball, baseball and other sports. It boasts a 71,168-seat stadium, several 18-hole golf courses, and other indoor and outdoor recreation facilities. Our location near a metropolitan area provides a strong primary and referral small animal case load. Columbia's proximity to rural central Missouri results in an exceptional food animal and equine case load.

> The unique curriculum gives students 2 years of undiluted clinical experience before graduation.

MU, a major research university with 33,000 students, consists of 18 schools and colleges located on a 1,262-acre campus. The College of Veterinary Medicine is noted for its unique curriculum that gives students nearly 2 years of clinical experience before graduation as opposed to the traditional 1-1.5 years. Students benefit from exposure to specialty medical areas such as clinical cardiology, neurology, orthopedics, ophthalmology, and oncology. Students also gain experience with advanced equipment such as a linear accelerator for treatment of cancer, MRI, state-of-the-art ultrasonography, extensive endoscopy equipment, cold lasers, a surgery room C-arm for radiography during surgical procedures, and others. MU is unique in having a medical school, nursing school, school of health-related professions, state cancer research center, the life sciences center, and department of animal science on the same campus, thus enhancing teaching, research, and clinical services.

APPLICATION INFORMATION

All applicants must apply through VMCAS and submit our Supplemental Application. For specific application information (availability, deadlines, fees, and VMCAS participation), please refer to the contact information listed above.

Residency implications: sixty seats are given to Missouri and sixty to non-residents. A total of 120 seats awarded each year. U.S. citizenship or permanent residency is required. Allows non-residents to gain residency after completing first year.

SUMMARY OF ADMISSION PROCEDURES

Mid-May 2017: VMCAS Application Opens.

August 1, 2017: Transcripts due to VMCAS.

VMCAS application and all letters of reference due: September 15, 2017 at 12 Midnight Eastern Time

Supplemental Missouri application due: September 16, 2017

Early January: Out-of-state interviews held. Must appear in person if invited.

February-March: Missouri interviews held.

Mid-April: Decisions mailed.

PREREQUISITES FOR ADMISSION

Course Description	Number of Hours/Credits	Necessity
English or Communication	6	Required
College algebra or higher	3	Required
Physics (complete sequence)	5	Required
Biological Science - not AS courses	10	Required
Humanities/Social Sciences	10	Required
Biochemistry with organic pre-req	3	Required
Electives	10	Required

Late August: Orientation and school begins.

ENTRANCE REQUIREMENTS

Required undergraduate GPA: Applicants must have a cumulative GPA of 3.00 or more on a 4.00 scale. The most recent entering class had a mean GPA of 3.77 at the time of acceptance.

AP credit policy: must appear on official college transcript and be equivalent to the appropriate college-level coursework.

Is a Bachelor's Degree Required? no

Is this an International School? no

ESTIMATED TUITION

Estimated Tuition Resident: $25,120

Estimated Tuition Contract: pending

Estimated Tuition Non-Resident: $54,192

AVAILABLE SEATS

Resident: 60

Contract: pending

Non-Resident: 60

TEST REQUIREMENTS

Standardized examinations: Graduate Record Examination (GRE) general test, including the analytical writing portion, must be completed within the last 3 years. A score of 285 (verbal and quantitative added together) and a 1.5 on the analytical is required. (Test must be taken after December 31, 2014 and submitted to VMCAS by September 15, 2017.)

VMCAS Participation: full

Accepts International Students? no

ADDITIONAL INFORMATION

Application Deadline: 9/15/2017

NORTH CAROLINA STATE UNIVERSITY

Email Address: cvm_dvm@ncsu.edu
Website: http://www.cvm.ncsu.edu

NC STATE UNIVERSITY | College of Veterinary Medicine

SCHOOL DESCRIPTION

The North Carolina State University College of Veterinary Medicine is located on a 182-acre site in Raleigh, the state capital, which has a population of more than 400,000. The sandy shores of North Carolina's beautiful coastline are a short ride to the east, and the Great Smoky Mountains are to the west. The climate includes mild winters and warm summers.

The College of Veterinary Medicine opened in the fall of 1981 and encompasses 20 buildings on the Centennial Biomedical Campus, including a teaching hospital, classrooms, animal wards, research and teaching laboratories, and health and wellness center, and working farm. The college has 150 faculty members and a capacity for 400 veterinary medical students with training for interns, residents, and graduate students.

> The College of Veterinary Medicine has 150 faculty members and a capacity for 400 veterinary medical students.

Construction started in fall 2002 on the Centennial Biomedical Campus, which is anchored by the College of Veterinary Medicine. An extension of the original NC State Centennial Campus concept, the Centennial Biomedical Campus will house approximately 30 building sites. It will include an additional 1.6 million square feet of space over the next 15 years, resulting in a five-fold expansion of the current college and veterinary health complex. The two-year construction of the Randall B. Terry, Jr. Companion Animal Veterinary Medical Center was completed in June 2011. The Terry Center is considered the national model for excellence in companion animal medicine.

The Terry Center offers cutting-edge technologies for imaging, cardiac care, cancer treatments, internal medicine, and surgery; has more than double the size of the former companion animal hospital; and accommodates the more than 27,000 cases referred to the CVM each year.

The Centennial Biomedical Campus emphasizes partnerships that work to bring academia, government and industry together. The focus of this campus is on biomedical applications, both to animals and humans. It provides opportunities for industry and government researchers, entrepreneurs, clinical trial companies, as well as collaborations with other universities to work side by side with faculty and students at the College of Veterinary Medicine.

APPLICATION INFORMATION

For specific application information (availability, deadlines, fees, and VMCAS participation), please refer to the contact information listed above.

Residency implications: priority is given to North Carolina residents. NOTE: The college increased its incoming class size from 80 to 100 starting with the 2012 admissions cycle. The current slot allocation is 80 resident and 20 non-resident slots. Non-resident admits are permitted to apply for residency for tuition purposes after the first 12 months in the program.

SUMMARY OF ADMISSION PROCEDURES

VMCAS application deadline: Friday, September 15, 2017 at 12 Midnight Eastern Time

PREREQUISITES FOR ADMISSION

Course Description	Number of Hours/Credits	Necessity
Animal Nutrition	3	Required
Biochemistry	3	Required
Biology	4	Required
Calculus or Logic	3	Required
Chemistry, General	8	Required
Chemistry, Organic	8	Required
Composition, Public Speaking or Communications	6	Required
Humanities and Social Sciences	6	Required
Microbiology	4	Required
Physics	8	Required
Statistics	3	Required
Genetics	4	Required

NC State Supplemental application deadline: Monday, September 18, 2017 at 1:00 PM Eastern Time

Date acceptances mailed: no later than April 1

School begins: August

Deposit (to hold place in class): $250.00

Deferments: are considered for 1 year only, subject to Admissions Committee approval

EVALUATION CRITERIA

Selection for admission is a 2-phase process.

Phase 1–Objective criteria:

Required course GPA: 3.3 Resident, 3.4 Nonresident

Cumulative GPA: 3.0 Resident, 3.4 Nonresident

Last 45 credit hour GPA: 3.3 Resident, 3.4 Nonresident

GRE test score

Supplemental Application

Phase 2–Subjective criteria:

1. Veterinary Experience
2. Animal Experience
3. Educational Experience
4. Evaluation Forms/Recommendations
5. Personal Statement
6. Diversity
7. Extracurricular and Community Activities

ENTRANCE REQUIREMENTS

AP credit policy: must appear on official college transcripts with course name and credit hours and be equivalent to the appropriate college-level coursework.

Is a Bachelor's Degree Required? no

Is this an International School? yes

ESTIMATED TUITION

Estimated Tuition Resident: $18,516

Estimated Tuition Contract: $0

Estimated Tuition Non-Resident: $43,753

AVAILABLE SEATS

Resident: 80

Contract: 0

Non-Resident: 20

TEST REQUIREMENTS

Standardized examinations: Graduate Record Examination (GRE), general test, is required. The scores must be received by the September 15th application deadline. There is no deadline to take the GRE.

VMCAS Participation: full

Accepts International Students? yes

ADDITIONAL INFORMATION

Application Deadline: 9/15/2017

THE OHIO STATE UNIVERSITY

Email Address: prospective@cvm.osu.edu
Website: www.vet.osu.edu/admissions

THE OHIO STATE UNIVERSITY

COLLEGE OF VETERINARY MEDICINE

SCHOOL DESCRIPTION

The Ohio State University is located in Columbus, the state's capital and the nation's 15th largest city. Columbus has been rated the 7th best city in the nation for cost of living (Forbes Magazine) and one of the country's top-10 places to live (Money). Columbus offers all the cultural perks you would expect from a major metropolitan area including the #1 zoo in the country, according to the USA Travel Guide.

The college is part of one of the largest and most comprehensive health sciences centers in the country.

The Ohio State University was founded in 1870 and is one of the nation's leading academic centers, consistently ranks as Ohio's best, and one of the nation's top-20 public universities. The campus consists of thousands of acres, hundreds of buildings, more than 15,000 faculty and staff, and more than 56,000 students.

The Veterinary Medical Center includes a Hospital for Companion Animals, Food Animal, and the Galbreath Equine Center. The patient load is one of the highest in the country and farmlands can be accessed 10 miles from campus. The Veterinary Medicine Academic Building has nearly 10,000 square feet of space and includes research labs, classrooms, a library, computer lab, and academic offices.

The Ohio State College of Veterinary Medicine is part of one of the largest and most comprehensive health sciences centers in the country that includes dentistry, medicine, nursing, optometry, pharmacy, public health, and veterinary medicine.

APPLICATION INFORMATION

For specific application information (availability, deadlines, fees, and VMCAS participation), please refer to the contact information listed above.

Residency implications: applicants from all states will be considered. In-state and out-of-state applicants are given equal consideration. We accept the top 162 students. We do accept international applicants.

SUMMARY OF ADMISSION PROCEDURES

VMCAS application deadline: Friday, September 15, 2017 at 12 Midnight Eastern Time

Date interviews are held: January

Date acceptances mailed: February-March

School begins: late August

Deposit (to hold place in class): $25.00 for residents; $325.00 (non-refundable fee) for non-resident applicants

Deferments: not considered

EVALUATION CRITERIA

General GRE, cumulative GPA, last 30 credit or semester hours and science GPA

Veterinary and animal experience (depth & diversity of experience)

Community/volunteer service, work and leadership experience

Letters of recommendation (Three are required at least one must be a veterinarian)

In-person interview

PREREQUISITES FOR ADMISSION

Course Description	Semester Hours (hours may vary)	Notes
Biochemistry*	4	If Biochemistry is taught as a 2-part sequence, both parts are required. Lab is not required.
Microbiology*	4	Lab is required.
Physiology**	5	All anatomy/physiology courses are taught as a 2-part sequence; both parts are required to fulfill this requirement. All systems must be covered. Lab is not required. Some schools may offer this as a combined Anatomy/Physiology course.
Public Speaking (Communication)	3	Basics of public speaking & critical thinking. This should be a public speaking course.
Science Electives	35	Includes, but not limited to: Biology, chemistry, anatomy, immunology, cell biology, molecular genetics, animal science, ecology, environmental science or other science courses.
Humanities/Social Science Electives	16	Includes, but not limited to: History, economics, anthropology, psychology, art, music, literature, languages, writing, and ethics.

* = Capstone Courses

**Physiology course work must be a comprehensive, intermediate systems physiology series. Required systems include musculoskeletal, neurology, urinary/renal, endocrine, reproductive, digestive, cardiovascular, and respiratory.

Science electives can include courses that are prerequisites for the capstone courses (e.g. biology, general and organic chemistry, etc.).

The number of hours provided is a guideline. In assessing course content for equivalency, actual hours may vary for your institution. In some cases a multiple course series may be needed to fulfill prerequisite coursework. If you are unsure of whether or not a course will be accepted to fulfill a prerequisite, please contact us at prospective@cvm.osu.edu.

Capstone courses - Biochemistry, Microbiology, Physiology, and Communication - must be completed with (1) a grade of C or better in each course, (2) a 3.0 (B) average among the courses, and (3) no more than one C between any of the four courses.

•If any of the capstone courses are taken as a multiple-part series, this rule will apply to each part as an individual course.

There may be additional courses that your school requires as prerequisites to the above courses. These additional courses can be used toward the elective requirements.

ADVANCED PLACEMENT

To receive credit for AP courses, they must be listed on official transcripts from a college or university you have attended.

Personal statement

Interview

Eligible applicants are interviewed and evaluated by members of the Admissions Committee.

ENTRANCE REQUIREMENTS

Required undergraduate GPA: the minimum GPA to be considered is 3.0 on a 4.0 scale. The most recent entering class had a mean overall GPA of 3.68 and a science GPA of 3.54. Science GPA is evaluated as well as last 30 semester or quarter hours.

AP credit policy: AP credit given if course is listed on official transcript.

Is a Bachelor's Degree Required? no

Is this an International School? no

COURSE COMPLETION DEADLINE

All of the prerequisite courses must be completed by the spring term preceding the autumn term when you would start vet school. (You do not have to have all of the prerequisites completed before applying.)

ESTIMATED TUITION

Estimated Tuition Resident: $31,150

Estimated Tuition Contract: $0

Estimated Tuition Non-Resident: $69,525

Tuition is subject to change.

*For tuition purposes, nonresident students can apply for residency after completing their first year at the Ohio State University.

AVAILABLE SEATS

Accept 162 students.

Resident: Up to 100

Contract: 0

Non-Resident: up to 80

TEST REQUIREMENTS

Standardized examinations: Graduate Record Examination (GRE) general test or the Medical College Admission (MCAT) test is required. Most applicants choose to take the GRE. Tests must be taken by September 1. Test scores must be received no later than September 15 of the year of application. GRE Code: 1592.

VMCAS Participation: full

Accepts International Students? yes

ADDITIONAL INFORMATION

Application Deadline: 9/15/2017

PRE-VETERINARY PROFILE: KAYLEE DEBUSK

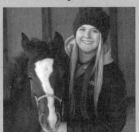

Current School Name
Washington State University

What type of veterinary medicine are you interested in pursuing, and why?
I am interested in pursuing equine medicine, possibly surgery. I grew up around horses and developed a love of working with them over the years.

What is/was your major during undergraduate school?
Animal science.

What are your short-term and long-term goals?
A short-term goal of mine is to finish the semester with a strong GPA, while a long-term goal of mine is to work at a reliable, ethical practice.

What are you doing as an applicant/pre-vet to prepare for veterinary school?
I have spent a large number of hours over the last five summers assisting a large animal vet. During this time, I have learned things that my classes haven't quite touched on yet. I have also learned what will be expected of me in vet school.

What extracurricular activities are you involved in currently?
I am a member of the WSU Women's Water Polo Club team. I also draw and paint regularly. Although I love school, it is nice to have hobbies that will serve as a mental break.

How old were you when you first became interested in being a veterinarian?
I was in middle school when I realized that I love horses, and I also love to fix things, which is part of what a career as a vet entails. If you have been around horses, you know that they can break down, so I knew that it would be a stable job that would give me satisfaction as well.

Please describe your various experiences in preparation for applying to veterinary school.
I had the fortune of meeting with a professor who is involved with the admissions at the WSU Vet school. I got to ask any personal questions that I had, and also got insight into what the admissions board is looking for in a student. Additionally, I have improved my organization and studying skills over the past few years, which I know will be a vital part of being a successful vet student.

What characteristics are you looking for in a veterinary school?
I am looking for a school that will allow its students to be as hands-on as possible and will give me the tools I need to have a good career.

What advice do you have for other pre-veterinary students?
I would say to not get discouraged. Yes, there will be a lot of schooling, and you will have to take a lot of tough classes, but if this is what you want to do, stick with it. If it were easy, everyone would do it.

OKLAHOMA STATE UNIVERSITY

Email Address: dvm@okstate.edu
Website: http://www.cvhs.okstate.edu

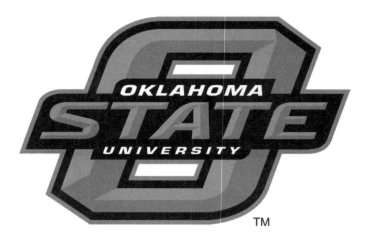

SCHOOL DESCRIPTION

Oklahoma State University is located in Stillwater, which has a population of about 46,000. Stillwater is in north central Oklahoma about 65 miles from Oklahoma City and 69 miles from Tulsa. The campus is exceptionally beautiful, with modified Georgian-style architecture in the new buildings. It encompasses 840 acres and more than 60 major academic buildings.

Three major buildings form the veterinary medicine complex. The oldest, McElroy Hall, houses the William E. Brock Memorial Library and Learning Center, as well as classrooms and laboratories. The Boren Veterinary Medical Teaching Hospital provides modern facilities for both academic and clinical instruction. Completing the triad is the Oklahoma Animal Disease Diagnostic Laboratory, which provides teaching resources for students in the professional curriculum and diagnostic services to Oklahoma agriculture and industry. The College of Veterinary Medicine is fully accredited by the American Veterinary Medical Association. Faculty members in the three academic departments share responsibility for the curriculum. These departments are Veterinary Clinical Sciences, Veterinary Pathobiology, and Physiological Sciences.

> Faculty members in the three OSU academic departments share responsibility for the curriculum.

APPLICATION INFORMATION

Residency implications: entering class size is 106, which includes 58 Oklahoma residents and 48 non-residents. A non-resident contract seat is available through AR.

SUMMARY OF ADMISSION PROCEDURES

Timetable

VMCAS application deadline: Friday, September 15, 2017 at 12 Midnight Eastern Time

Date interviews held: February

Date acceptances mailed: March

School begins: mid-August

Deposit (to hold place in class): resident, $100.00; non-resident, $500.00

EVALUATION CRITERIA

The admission procedure consists of evaluation of both academic and nonacademic criteria. The Admissions Committee considers all factors in the applicant's file, but the following are especially important: academic achievement; familiarity with the profession and sincerity of interest; recommendations; test scores; extracurricular activities; character, personality, and commitment for a career in veterinary medicine. The committee selects those applicants considered most capable of excelling as veterinary medical students and who possess the greatest potential for success in the veterinary medical profession.

PREREQUISITES FOR ADMISSION

Course Description	Minimum Number of Hours/Credits	Necessity
Animal Nutrition	3	Required
Biochemistry	3	Required
Biology/Zoology	8	Required
English, Speech, or Composition	9	Required
Genetics	3	Required
Humanities/Social Science	6	Required
Inorganic Chemistry	8	Required
Math (College Algebra - No Statistics)	3	Required
Microbiology	4	Required
Organic Chemistry (5-hour survey accepted)	8	Required
Physics 1 & 2	8	Required

ENTRANCE REQUIREMENTS

Required undergraduate GPA: a minimum GPA of 2.8 (on a 4.0 scale) is required in prerequisite courses. The mean cumulative GPA of the 2016 entering class was 3.609.

AP credit policy: AP credit accepted if documented on college transcript.

Is a Bachelor's Degree Required? no

Is this an International School? no

ESTIMATED TUITION

Estimated Tuition Resident: $20,780 (tuition + fees for one full year)

Estimated Tuition Contract: $0

Estimated Tuition Non-Resident: 45,890 (tuition + fees for one full year)

AVAILABLE SEATS

Resident: 58

Contract: 0

Non-Resident: 48

TEST REQUIREMENTS

Standardized examinations: Graduate Record Examination (GRE), general test is required. The class of 2020 had mean scores of 153 verbal, 152 quantitative, and analytical of 4.0. Scores must be sent to code 6558 by October 15.

VMCAS Participation: full

Accepts International Students? yes

ADDITIONAL INFORMATION

Application Deadline: 9/15/2017

OREGON STATE UNIVERSITY

Email Address: cvmadmissions@oregonstate.edu
Website: www.oregonstate.edu/vetmed

SCHOOL DESCRIPTION

Oregon State University is located in Corvallis, the heart of the Willamette Valley. Our climate is mild year-round, with ocean beaches less than an hour drive to the west and some of the best snow skiing in the Cascade Range a little over two hours to the east. Major metropolitan attractions can be found less than two hours away in Eugene, Salem and Portland. Corvallis has a population of approximately 55,000 and is a beautiful and friendly place to live and pursue your education.

> Hands-on education is an important aspect to how our students learn and develop knowledge of the profession.

The Oregon State University College of Veterinary Medicine has the smallest class size of the DVM programs in the U.S., admitting only 72 students per year. Hands-on education is an important aspect to how our students learn and develop their knowledge of the profession. Our partnership with the Oregon Humane Society provides an opportunity for students to continue acquiring skills and confidence in their ability to perform as professionals. Students at OSU work in state-of-the-art facilities alongside our world-class faculty, including specialists in cardiology, oncology, imaging, and rehabilitation. The individual attention our students get from faculty and hospital staff is, in part, why year after year nearly 100% percent of our students pass their board exams.

APPLICATION INFORMATION

All components of the Oregon State DVM application are due by September 15. No materials will be accepted after this date including transcripts and GRE scores.

SUMMARY OF ADMISSION PROCEDURES

Steps to apply for admission to Oregon State University College of Veterinary Medicine:
1. Begin the VMCAS application process
2. Request all transcripts be sent direct to VMCAS, they must be received by September 15, 2017.
   VMCAS Transcripts
   P O Box 9126
   Watertown, MA 02471
3. Submit GRE scores directly to VMCAS using the directions provided on their website.
4. Complete VMCAS with electronic letters of recommendation
5. Complete Oregon State University supplemental application by September 15, 2017 at 12 Midnight Eastern Time.
6. Pay online supplemental application fee of $50.00

ENTRANCE REQUIREMENTS

All pre-requisites for OSU must be completed with a grade of C- or better.

Is a Bachelor's Degree Required? no

Is this an International School? yes

PREREQUISITES FOR ADMISSION

Course Description	Number of Hours/Credits	Necessity
General Biology I	3	Required
General Biology II	3	Required
Upper Division Biology w/ Lab	4	Required
Physics I	4	Required
Physics II	4	Required
General Chemistry I w/ Lab	4	Required
General Chemistry II w/ Lab	4	Required
Organic Chemistry I	3	Required
Biochemistry I	4	Required
Genetics	3	Required
Calculus or Algebra & Trig	4	Required
Statistics	3	Required
Physiology (Human or Animal)	3	Required
English	4	Required
Humanities or Social Sciences	8	Required
Public Speaking	3	Required

Please note that the General Education Requirements (English, Humanities, & Public Speaking) will be considered met if the applicant has earned a bachelor's degree by July 1 of the year in which they are accepted into the program.

ESTIMATED TUITION

Estimated Tuition Resident: $23,079

Estimated Tuition Contract: $23,079 plus additional $4,000 per year scholarship

Estimated Tuition Non-Resident: $44,589

AVAILABLE SEATS

Resident: 40

Non-Resident (including Contract positions): 32

TEST REQUIREMENTS

VMCAS Participation: full

Accepts International Students? yes

ADDITIONAL INFORMATION

Conversion for quarter credits of our pre-requisites is available on our website.

Application Deadline: 9/15/2017

UNIVERSITY OF PENNSYLVANIA

Email Address: admissions@vet.upenn.edu
Website: www.vet.upenn.edu

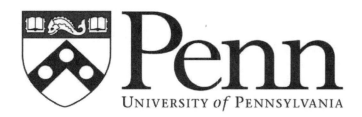

SCHOOL DESCRIPTION

The University of Pennsylvania is located in West Philadelphia. Philadelphia is a city with a strong cultural heritage. Independence National Park includes 1 square mile of historic Philadelphia next to the Delaware River. Included are Independence Hall, the Liberty Bell, and many fine examples of colonial architecture. Philadelphia also offers theaters, museums, sports, and outdoor recreation. The Philadelphia Zoo, first in the nation, houses more than 1,600 mammals, birds, reptiles, and amphibians.

> The School of Veterinary Medicine enjoys a close relationship with the Philadelphia zoo, first in the nation.

The School of Veterinary Medicine enjoys a close relationship with the zoo. The School of Veterinary Medicine was founded in 1884 and includes a hospital for small animals, classrooms, and research facilities in the city. The large-animal hospital and research facilities are located at the New Bolton Center, an 800-acre farm 40 miles west of Philadelphia. The first 2 years are spent on the main campus. Part of the third year may be spent at the New Bolton Center, and the fourth year is spent in rotation and on electives at varying campus locations. Off-campus electives are frequently permitted.

APPLICATION INFORMATION

For specific application information (availability, deadlines, fees, and VMCAS participation), please refer to the contact information listed above.

Residency implications: priority is given to Pennsylvania residents. The number of nonresident places is usually about 85, including international applicants.

2015-2016 admissions summary for the class of 2020:

	Number of Applicants	Number of Entrants
Resident	206	50
Non-Resident	888	73
Total	1,194	123

SUMMARY OF ADMISSION PROCEDURES

Timetable

VMCAS application deadline: Friday, September 15, 2017 at 12 Midnight Eastern Time

Supplemental application and fee deadline: September 15

Date interviews are held: Fridays from early January until completion

Date acceptances mailed: within 14 days after interview

School begins: early September

Deposit (to hold place in class): $500.00

Deferments: are considered on an individual basis.

EVALUATION CRITERIA

The seats are filled through a 2-part admission procedure, which includes a file review and personal interviews.

Grades

Test scores

Animal/veterinary experience

PREREQUISITES FOR ADMISSION

Course Description	Number of Hours/Credits
English (including composition)	6
Physics (with lab)	8
Chemistry - General (with at least 1 lab)	8
Chemistry - Organic	4
Biology or Zoology (covering basic genetics & cell bio)	9
Biochem	3
Microbiology	3
Social sciences or humanities	6
Calculus & Statistics (Any Introductory Stats course)	6
Electives	37

Interview

References

Essay

English skills (TOEFL)

File review: files are reviewed in late Fall by members of the admissions committee (including an alumni member), and decisions are made on whether or not to offer an interview.

Personal interviews: interviews are held on Fridays from early January until the class is filled. The number of interviews granted equals approximately 2 times the number of seats available.

Two personal interviews are conducted: a formal interview with 1 member of the Admissions Committee and 1 observer from the auxiliary interviewer pool on Admissions, and an informal interview with student committee members. Although students do not vote on acceptance, they have a significant part in the meeting following interviews.

ENTRANCE REQUIREMENTS

Required undergraduate GPA: no specific GPA. Applicants are evaluated comparatively. The mean cumulative GPA of the class admitted in 2016 was 3.59.

AP credit policy: must appear on official college transcripts and count toward degree.

Course completion deadline: All prerequisite courses must be completed by the end of the 1st Summer Session of the year in which admission is sought.

ADDITIONAL REQUIREMENTS/CONSIDERATIONS

Animal/veterinary work experience: experience working with animals, direct veterinary work, or research experience is desired. Approximately 500-600 hours is recommended. Experience should be sufficient to convince the admissions committee of motivation, interest, and understanding.

Recommendations/evaluations: 3 required, one from an academic science source; and one from a veterinarian. The third is the choice of the applicant.

Extracurricular/community service activities: additional activities in this category can provide information important to the admissions committee.

Leadership: evidence of leadership abilities is desirable.

Is a Bachelor's Degree Required? no

Is this an International School? no

ESTIMATED TUITION

Estimated Tuition and Fees Resident: $45,798

Estimated Tuition and Fees Contract: Not Applicable

Estimated Tuition and Fees Non-Resident: $55,798

AVAILABLE SEATS

Resident: 40

Contract: Not Applicable

Non-Resident: 85

TEST REQUIREMENTS

Standardized examinations: Graduate Record Examination (GRE), general test, is required; the GRE Code for Pennvet is 2775. Test scores should be received no later than September 15.

VMCAS Participation: full

Accepts International Students? yes

ADDITIONAL INFORMATION

Dual-Degree Programs: Combined VMD-graduate degree programs are available.

Summer Program: Penn Vet offers a summer program for high school and college students. The Veterinary Exploration Through Science (VETS) program, now in its eighth year is a day program of one-week sessions designed for those who want a close-up look at veterinary medicine. For additional information, please visit our website at www.vet.upenn.edu/education /admissions/summer-vets-program or call 215-898-5434.

Application Deadline: 9/15/2017

PURDUE UNIVERSITY

Email Address: vetadmissions@purdue.edu
Website: http://www.vet.purdue.edu
Phone: 765-494-7893

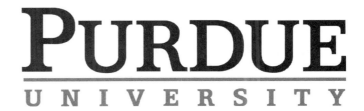

INDIANA

SCHOOL DESCRIPTION

Purdue University is located in one of the largest metropolitan centers in northwestern Indiana. Greater Lafayette occupies a site on the Wabash River 65 miles northwest of Indianapolis and 126 miles southeast of Chicago. The combined population of the twin cities, Lafayette and West Lafayette, exceeds 100,000. The community offers an art museum, historical museum, 1,600 acres of public parks, and more than 60 churches of all major denominations.

> Purdue emphasizes the veterinary team approach, problem solving, and hands-on experiences.

Purdue ranks among the 25 largest colleges and universities in the nation. Students represent all 50 states and many foreign countries. Purdue University has the third highest enrollment of international students of any college in the United States. The Purdue University College of Veterinary Medicine strives to become the leading veterinary school for comprehensive education of the veterinary team and for discovery and engagement in selected areas of veterinary and comparative biomedical sciences. To better prepare individuals for veterinary medical careers in the twenty-first century, our curriculum emphasizes the veterinary team approach, problem-solving, and hands-on experiences.

APPLICATION INFORMATION

For specific application information, please refer to the contact information listed above.

Each veterinary class has 84 students. The class will be seated with approximately 50% residents and 50% non-resident students.

SUMMARY OF ADMISSION PROCEDURES

Timetable

VMCAS application deadline: Friday, September 15, 2017 at 12 Midnight Eastern Time

Date interviews are held: January

Date acceptances released: February

Classes begin: late August

Deposit (to hold place in class): $400.00 for residents; $1,000.00 for nonresidents. Deposit applied to tuition after matriculation.

Deferments: request for deferments will be considered on a case-by-case basis.

EVALUATION CRITERIA

The admission process consists of:

A preliminary review based upon grade point indices, test scores, and prerequisite course completion

An in-depth review of selected applicants

A personal interview by invitation is required

% Weight

Grades, overall academic performance - 55% weight (including academic rigor)

Animal, veterinary, research, and general work experiences, extracurricular activities, leadership, personal

PREREQUISITES FOR ADMISSION		
Course Description	Semester(s)	Necessity
General (Inorganic) Chemistry with Lab I	1	Required
General (Inorganic) Chemistry with Lab II	1	Required
Organic Chemistry with Lab I	1	Required
Organic Chemistry with Lab II	1	Required
Biochemistry (upperlevel)	1	Required
General Biology with Lab I	1	Required
General Biology with Lab II	1	Required
Genetics	1	Required
Microbiology with Lab	1	Required
Animal Nutrition	1	Required
Physics with Lab I	1	Required
Physics with Lab II	1	Required
Statistics	1	Required
English Composition	1	Required
Communication	1	Required
Humanities	3	Required

statement, overall presentation of application materials, honors and awards, references, and interview - 45% weight

ENTRANCE REQUIREMENTS

Required undergraduate GPA: the mean cumulative GPA of the entering class in the fall of 2016 for resident students was 3.62 on a 4.00 scale and for non-resident students was 3.62 on a 4.00 scale. The minimum cumulative GPA required for consideration is 3.00 on a 4.00 scale.

AP credit policy: will be accepted if it appears on official college transcripts by subject area and is equivalent to the appropriate college-level coursework. Should your institution's official transcript not list the subject area, then you may submit an unofficial transcript with a letter explaining this and indicating which prerequisite courses are met by these credits.

Is a Bachelor's Degree Required? no

Is this an International School? no

ESTIMATED TUITION

Estimated Tuition Resident: $19,928

Estimated Tuition Contract: n/a

Estimated Tuition Non-Resident: $44,756

AVAILABLE SEATS

Resident: 42

Contract: 0

Non-Resident: 42

TEST REQUIREMENTS

Standardized examinations: none

VMCAS Participation: full

Accepts International Students? yes

ADDITIONAL INFORMATION:

Application Deadline: 9/15/2017

FIRST-YEAR PROFILE: MIKE MANNEBACH

Current School Name
Virginia-Maryland College of Veterinary Medicine

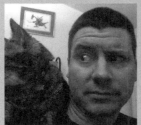

Why do you want to be a veterinarian?
Holding a sleeping pet in your lap—utterly vulnerable, yet completely at ease—you realize just how deep their trust is. It can be a humbling experience. They have a sort of fundamental innocence, relying on us for their safety and well-being, and trusting that we will provide it. Veterinarians help pet owners fulfill their side of that unspoken agreement. They help people better understand their pet, and thereby enhance the bond between them. They help keep pets healthy, increasing the time we have with them. At the end, they allow the pet owner to give their loved one a final gift: relief from suffering and fear, and a graceful exit from this world. That work is inherently meaningful—it is work I want to do.

What are your short-term and long-term goals?
I would like to survive vet school and earn my degree, mastering the fundamental knowledge and skills that will enable me to be the best doctor I can be. After graduation, I hope to work in a small animal clinic with several experienced doctors. Every veterinarian I've worked with has taught me something, and each one has a unique perspective. As I begin my career caring for pets (and their owners), I will look to the experience and guidance of those doctors to continue my own growth and aptitude. I also look forward to developing relationships with clients. The bond between people and their pets is powerful and beautiful; it will be a privilege to play even a small part in strengthening that bond. Longer-term, my only goal is honest reflection about what I want and need from my career. Right now, I would love to return to vet school someday as an instructor. Only time will tell whether the 10-years-from-now me has those same aspirations.

What did you do as an applicant to prepare for applying to veterinary school?
I got help. The staff at VMCAS were fantastic about demystifying the application process and providing a timeline of what needed to be done and when. The admissions team at VMCVM was terrific, helping to untangle the list of prerequisites, and setting my mind at ease that I had each of them covered. My doctors and professors were very generous with their time and effort in writing my letters of recommendation. Ultimately, it is your own responsibility to make sure your application is complete and on time. However, that doesn't mean you have to do it completely alone.

What advice would you give to applicants or those considering applying to veterinary school?
Be sure—really sure—that it's what you want. Work with, shadow, and talk to vets who are living the career you want; ask them about the difficult, unpleasant, challenging parts of their work. Vet school is just too large an investment of money, time, opportunity-cost, and stress to take on, with anything less than complete confidence in your decision.

What helped make the transition to veterinary school easier for you?
The support of family, friends, and co-workers. I'm amazingly fortunate to have so many people I love and respect, all speaking with one voice: "You can do it!" My work experience (this is my second career) has also eased the transition. I've been in positions that expected 50-60 hour work weeks, and for several years my normal work schedule was Monday to Saturday. Even with that experience, my first semester of vet school is the most challenging thing I've ever done, but at least I'm tackling it, confident that I can dedicate the study time, and sustain the pace.

What is your advice on student debt?
I have no advice of my own, but here are three things I've been told, all of which ring strongly true: 1) Minimize your debt as much as you can. If you get accepted to your in-state vet school, go there. Live as frugally as possible. If you own a functional car/laptop/phone/whatever, don't replace it with a shiny new (expensive) one. 2) Prepare yourself mentally to live like a broke college student—even for many years after you graduate. 3) Educate yourself politically and vote for candidates (at all levels of government) who recognize the growing student debt crisis and who support policies that provide relief from it.

UNIVERSITY OF TENNESSEE

Email Address: dshepherd@utk.edu
Website: http://www.vet.utk.edu

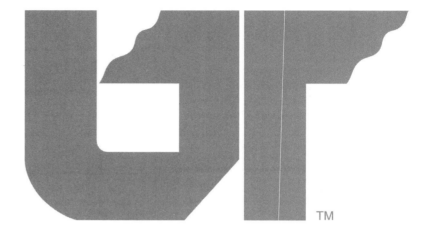

SCHOOL DESCRIPTION

The University of Tennessee's College of Veterinary Medicine is located in Knoxville, a city of 185,000 situated in the Appalachian foothills of east central Tennessee. Only 45 minutes from the Great Smoky Mountains National Park and 3 hours from both Nashville and Atlanta, Knoxville offers many recreational and cultural opportunities, including a symphony orchestra, an opera company, and several fine theaters. The climate in Knoxville is moderate with distinct seasons.

The Knoxville campus of the University of Tennessee has about 21,300 undergraduate and 6,200 graduate students.

The 550-acre Knoxville campus of the University of Tennessee has about 21,300 undergraduate and 6,200 graduate students. The modern Clyde M. York Veterinary Medicine Building, housing the teaching and research facilities, the Veterinary Medical Center, including the W.W. Armistead Veterinary Teaching Hospital, and Agriculture-Veterinary Medicine Library, faces the Tennessee River on the university's Agricultural Campus.

The curriculum of the College of Veterinary Medicine is a 9-semester, 4-year program. Development of a strong basic science education is emphasized in the first year. The second and third years emphasize the study of diseases, their causes, diagnosis, treatment, and prevention. Innovative features of the first three years of the curriculum include 6 weeks of student-centered small-group applied-learning exercises in semesters 1-5; 3 weeks of dedicated clinical experiences in the Veterinary Medical Center in semesters 3-5; and elective course opportunities in semesters 4-9 that allow students to focus on specific educational/ career goals. In the fourth year (final 3 semesters), students participate exclusively in clinical rotations (27 weeks of core rotations and 23 weeks of elective rotations) in the Veterinary Medical Center and in required off-campus externships. The college has unique programs in zoo, avian, and exotic animal medicine and surgery, cancer diagnosis and therapy, minimally invasive surgery (laser lithotripsy, endoscopy, otoscopy), and rehabilitation/physical therapy.

APPLICATION INFORMATION

For specific application information (availability, deadlines, fees, and VMCAS participation), please refer to the contact information listed above. We admit approximately 85 applicants each year. Priority is given to Tennessee residents (60 of the 85 seats are for Tennessee residents). Twenty-five highly qualified non-residents are admitted each year.

Residency implications: Tennessee has no contractual agreements for residency waivers. Tennessee accepts applications from United States citizens and permanent residents of the United States. Applications from international students completing the recognized prerequisites will be considered for 2017. TOEFL score and international student requirements can be found at http://international.utk.edu.

SUMMARY OF ADMISSION PROCEDURES

Timetable

VMCAS application deadline: Friday, September 15, 2017 at 12 Midnight Eastern Time

PREREQUISITES FOR ADMISSION

Course	Credits
General inorganic chemistry (with laboratory)	8
Organic chemistry (with laboratory)	8
General biology/zoology (with laboratory)	8
Cellular/Molecular biology*	3
Genetics	3
Biochemistry (exclusive of laboratory)†	4
Physics (with laboratory)	8
English composition	6
Social sciences/humanities	18

* It is expected that this requirement will be fulfilled by a course in cellular or molecular biology. An upper-division cell or molecular biology course is preferred.

† This should be a complete upper-division course in general cellular and comparative biochemistry. Half of a 2-semester sequence will not satisfy this requirement. Applicants are strongly encouraged to complete additional biological and physical science courses, especially comparative anatomy, mammalian physiology, microbiology with laboratory, and statistics.

GRE scores must be received no later than September 15, 2017

Date interviews are held: TBD in January 2018

Date acceptances mailed: the week of February 19, 2018

Applicant's response date: April 16, 2018

School begins: mid-August 2018

Deposit (to hold place in class): none required.

Deferments: are considered on a case-by-case basis.

EVALUATION CRITERIA

The admission procedure consists of a 3-phased review process (i.e., academic review, packet review, and interview). Each section weighted equally in the final applicant score. The initial academic review determines which applicants will move forward to a packet review. The combined academic review and packet review determines selection of the applicant interview pool.

Initial academic file review includes:
Academic performance and grade point average
GRE Test scores
Prerequisite completion
VMCAS and Supplemental Application information
VMCAS Disadvantaged/Hardship statement (optional)

Holistic packet review:
Rigor of educational program and potential for success
Personal Statement
References (3-5 required – 3 veterinarian letters preferred)
Evidence of logical preparation for this career
Veterinary and Animal Experience
Extracurricular activities/community service
Leadership and diversity
Disadvantaged/Hardship factors

Interview:
Personal Statement
Animal/veterinary experience
Communication skills
Motivation
Understanding of the profession
Personal interests and qualities
Professionalism

ENTRANCE REQUIREMENTS

Required undergraduate GPA: for nonresident applicants, the minimum acceptable cumulative GPA is 3.20 on a 4.00 scale. At time of acceptance, the mean GPA of the class entering in fall of 2016 was 3.59.

AP credit policy: must appear on official college transcripts and be equivalent to the appropriate college-level coursework.

Course completion deadline: prerequisite courses must be completed with a grade of C or better by the end of the spring term prior to entry.

Is a Bachelor's Degree Required? no

Is this an International School? no

ESTIMATED TUITION

Estimated Tuition Resident: $28,428

Estimated Tuition Contract: $0

Estimated Tuition Non-Resident: $56,500

AVAILABLE SEATS

Resident: 60

Contract: 0

Non-Resident: 25

TEST REQUIREMENTS

Standardized examinations: Graduate Record Exam (GRE), General Test (Verbal, Quantitative, and Analytical) is required, and scores must be received by September 15, 2017. (To assure scores are reported by the application deadline, applicants should consider exam dates prior to August 15, 2017.)

English Language Requirement: Applicants whose native language is not English are required to take and pass the Test of English as a Foreign Language (TOEFL) or the International English Language Testing System (IELTS). Passing marks are 550, 213, 80, and 6.5 for paper-based, computer-based, internet-based (iBT) TOEFL, and IELTS respectively. Official scores must be received directly from the appropriate testing service. TOEFL scores must be received by Jan. 25, 2018.

The University of Tennessee's score reporting code for TOEFL is 1843. The score must not be older than two years from the requested date of entry. Applicants who have received a degree from an accredited US institution in the past two years are exempt from the TOEFL or IELTS requirement.

TOEFL information may be obtained from the official TOEFL website.

IELTS information may be obtained from the official IELTS website.

VMCAS Participation: full

Accepts International Students? yes

ADDITIONAL INFORMATION

Additional requirements and considerations:
Animal/veterinary work experience
3 letters of recommendation are required but no more than 5 letters will be accepted. Two should be from veterinarians.
Extracurricular and/community service activities
Leadership skills
Autobiographical essay (personal statement)
A Supplemental Application is required and an optional Disadvantages Declaration and can be found at: http://www.vet.utk.edu/admissions/supplemental

Dual Degree Program
The College, in partnership with the College of Education, Health and Human Sciences, offers an option for veterinary students (and graduate veterinarians) to earn the MPH degree with a concentration in Veterinary Public Health.

Contact the College of Veterinary Medicine, Dr. Marcy Souza at msouza@utk.edu for additional information.

Dual DVM/PhD Program
The College, in partnership with the Graduate School, offers a dual DVM/PhD program option to students interested in a research career. Students are eligible to take a limited number of courses to count toward a PhD degree in Comparative and Experimental Medicine. Entry to the program requires a separate application to the graduate school. For more information visit http://www.vet.utk.edu/graduate/index.php

*Please see our website for complete information at: https://vetmed.tennessee.edu/admissions/Pages/admissions -process.aspx

TEXAS A&M UNIVERSITY

Email Address: studentadmissions@cvm.tamu.edu
Website: http://vetmed.tamu.edu

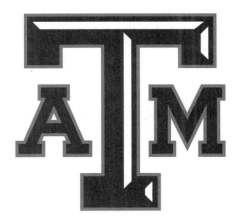

SCHOOL DESCRIPTION

The university is located adjacent to the cities of Bryan and College Station. The two cities have a combined population of approximately 200,000. The student population at Texas A&M is more than 58,000. The College of Veterinary Medicine is one of the 10 original veterinary teaching institutions that existed in the United States prior to World War II.

The College provides an integrated professional curriculum that prepares graduates with a firm foundation in the basic sciences, a broad comparative medicine knowledge base, and the clinical and personal skills to be leaders in the many career fields of veterinary medicine. Professional students are given the opportunity to gain additional education and training in their personal career paths.

> The College of Veterinary Medicine is one of the 10 original teaching institutions that existed in the US prior to World War II.

Becoming a veterinarian requires much dedication and diligent study. The veterinary medical student is required to meet a high level of performance. The demands on students' time and effort are considerable, but the rewards and career satisfaction are personal achievements that make significant contributions to our society.

APPLICATION INFORMATION

For specific application information (availability, deadlines and fees), please refer to the contact information listed above.

Residency implications: Texas has no contractual agreements with other states. Applicants from other states who have outstanding credentials will be considered. Texas seats 130 residents and up to 10 non-resident applicants per year. In the event that not all 10 non-resident positions are filled, these positions will then be filled with Texas alternates. Successful non-resident candidates who are awarded competitive university-based scholarships may attend at the resident tuition rate.

SUMMARY OF ADMISSION PROCEDURES

Timetable

Application deadline: September 30

Date interviews are held: mid-January

Date acceptances mailed: mid-March

School begins: late August

Deposit (to hold place in class): none required

Deferments: requests for deferments will be considered on a case-by-case basis

EVALUATION CRITERIA

Academic performance

Test scores

Interview

Personal statement

Evaluations (3 evaluations are required. 1 evaluation must be from a veterinarian with whom you have worked with. No letters of support/recommendation are needed)

PREREQUISITES FOR ADMISSION		
Course Description	Number of Hours/Credits	Necessity
General Biology with lab	4	Required
General Microbiology with lab	4	Required
Genetics	3	Required
Animal Nutrition or Feeds & Feeding	3	Required
Inorganic Chemistry I & II with lab	8	Required
Organic Chemistry I & II with lab	8	Required
Biochemistry (lecture hours only)	3	Required
Statistics (upper level)	3	Required
Physics I & II with lab	8	Required
Composition & Rhetoric	3	Required
Introduction to Psychology	3	Required
Technical Writing	3	Required
Speech Communication	3	Required

Semester course load and post-academic challenge

Leadership and experience

ENTRANCE REQUIREMENTS

Required undergraduate GPA: the minimum overall GPA required is 2.90 on a 4.00 scale and 3.10 for the last 45 GPA and 2.90 Science GPA. The mean of the most recent entering class was 3.68.

AP credit policy: AP credit is accepted as fulfilling selected prerequisites; credit must be reflected on the official undergraduate transcript.

Is a Bachelor's Degree Required? no

Is this an International School? no

ESTIMATED TUITION

Estimated Tuition Resident: $22,470

Estimated Tuition Contract: $0

Estimated Tuition Non-Resident: $33,868

AVAILABLE SEATS

Resident: 130

Contract: 0

Non-Resident: 10

TEST REQUIREMENTS

Standardized examinations: Graduate Record Examination (GRE), general test, is required. Beginning August 1, 2011, the College of Veterinary Medicine will require the new version of the GRE examination. Deadline for taking the GRE will be September 30. Scores over 5 years old will not be accepted.

VMCAS Participation: non-VMCAS

Accepts International Students? no

ADDITIONAL INFORMATION

Application Deadline: 9/29/2017 (5 p.m. CST)

TUFTS UNIVERSITY

Email Address: vetadmissions@tufts.edu
Website: http://vet.tufts.edu

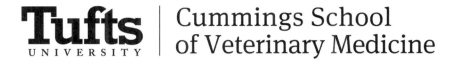

Cummings School
of Veterinary Medicine

SCHOOL DESCRIPTION

Cummings School of Veterinary Medicine at Tufts University is committed to advancing One Health initiatives that enhance the health and well-being of animals, humans and the environment. Cummings School is well-positioned to apply One Health philosophies, leveraging the collective expertise of Tufts University's constellation of health science schools, including veterinary, medical, dental, and nutrition. The University's leadership in both clinical and research settings reaches across disciplines, into the classroom, and out into the world.

> Tufts' leadership in clinical and research settings reaches across disciplines, into the classroom, and into the world.

Our faculty advance science, improve patient care and, most importantly, inspire our students to approach their profession with open minds and a desire to make a difference. The relatively small student body ensures close professional relationships and networking opportunities. An array of curricular options, including electives and dual degree programs, allows each student to find and nurture his or her evolving niche within the profession.

Veterinary students play an integral role in the seven hospitals and clinics that comprise Cummings Veterinary Medical Center at Tufts. From their first year onward, students gain valuable expertise and enjoy a rich clinical learning environment at the:

- Foster Hospital for Small Animals, offering one of the largest small animal caseloads in the country, especially in the area of emergency and critical care where we are designated by the American College of Veterinary Emergency and Critical Care as a national Veterinary Trauma Center.
- Lerner Spay and Neuter Clinic, where students hone their surgical skills.
- Hospital for Large Animals, providing active involvement in the diagnosis, treatment and prevention of disease in horses, especially equine athletes and sport horses, camelids and small ruminants.
- Wildlife Clinic, engaging students in the hands-on practice of wildlife medicine as well as the larger ethical and conservation issues that impact wildlife, people, and the environment.
- Tufts at Tech Community Veterinary Clinic, an innovative, low-cost clinic located within a public technical high school, where students provide primary care to underserved communities in the area.
- Tufts Ambulatory Service, the largest food animal practice in southern New England, addressing health and production needs of cattle, small ruminants and horses. The School's farm, just steps away from the classroom, offers additional hands-on experience in agriculture and food supply veterinary medicine.
- Tufts Veterinary Emergency Treatment and Specialties (Tufts VETS), providing students the opportunity to work in an after-hours urgent care and specialty setting that closely aligns with a private practice business model.

PREREQUISITES FOR ADMISSION

Course Description	Number of Hours/Credits	Necessity
Biology with laboratory	8	Required
Chemistry with laboratory	8	Required
Organic Chemistry with laboratory	8	Required
Biochemistry	3	Required
Physics	6	Required
Genetics*	3	Required
Mathematics/Statistics	6	Required
English/Speech	6	Required
Humanities and Fine Arts	6	Required
Social and Behavioral Sciences	6	Required

* unless included in biology

Students engage in a myriad of opportunities, including basic, translational and clinical research, shelter medicine, comparative oncology, wildlife and conservation medicine, the study of human-animal interactions, regenerative medicine, and more. A major international grant, Emerging Pandemic Threats One Health Workforce, and the International Veterinary Medicine certificate program, along with other ongoing projects, allow students to contribute to global One Health. These opportunities create a campus without boundaries, offer unique learning experiences, and ultimately lead our graduates to exciting and fulfilling careers.

Located just 30 miles west of the city of Boston, students take advantage of the area's internationally renowned teaching hospitals and biomedical research centers, as well as join in the vibrant atmosphere of more than 300,000 college students living, learning, and growing together.

We invite you to explore our web site and visit our campus to learn more about Cummings School of Veterinary Medicine at Tufts University: vet.tufts.edu.

APPLICATION INFORMATION

For specific application information (availability, deadlines, fees, and VMCAS participation), please refer to the contact information listed above.

Residency implications: Massachusetts residents make up about one-third of each class.

SUMMARY OF ADMISSION PROCEDURES

Timetable

VMCAS Application Deadline: Friday, September 15, 2017 at 12 Midnight Eastern Time

Date interviews are held: December, January, February

Date acceptances mailed: March

School begins: late August

Deposit (to hold place in class): $500.00

Deferments: requests for deferment are handled on a case-by-case basis.

EVALUATION CRITERIA

Tufts' admission procedure consists of a review of the application and an interview of selected applicants.

ENTRANCE REQUIREMENTS

Required undergraduate GPA: no minimum GPA required. The mean GPA for the Class of 2020 was 3.67.

AP credit policy: must appear on official college transcripts and be equivalent to the appropriate college-level coursework.

Is a Bachelor's Degree Required? no

Is this an International School? no

ESTIMATED TUITION

Estimated Tuition Resident: $48,890

Estimated Tuition Contract: N/A

Estimated Tuition Non-Resident: $53,957

AVAILABLE SEATS

Resident: 30

Contract: 0

Non-Resident: 68

TEST REQUIREMENTS

Standardized examinations: Graduate Record Examinations (GRE), general test, is required. The most recent acceptable test date for applicants to the class of 2021 is September 15, 2017. Scores are valid for five years. The mean GRE scores for the Class of 2020 were: Verbal 161, Quantitative 159, and Analytical Writing 4.5.

VMCAS Participation: full

Accepts International Students? yes

ADDITIONAL INFORMATION

Application Deadline: 9/15/2017

TUSKEGEE UNIVERSITY

Website: http://www.onemedicine.tuskegee.edu/CVM_TU/ac

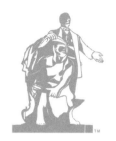

TUSKEGEE

UNIVERSITY

SCHOOL DESCRIPTION

Tuskegee University College of Veterinary Medicine is located in Tuskegee, Alabama, a city of about 13,000. Tuskegee is 40 miles east of the state of Alabama, Capitol City, Montgomery, and twenty miles west of the city of Auburn. It is also within easy driving distance to the cities of Birmingham, Alabama and Atlanta, Georgia. Summers are hot with moderate to mild humidity, and winters are moderate. Its recreational facilities, lakes, and parks can be enjoyed throughout the year-round.

> The University stresses the need to educate the whole person, that is, the hand and the heart as well as the mind.

Since it was founded by Booker T. Washington in 1881, Tuskegee University (HBCU) has become one of our nation's most outstanding institutions of higher learning. While it focuses on helping to develop human resources primarily within the African-American community, it is open to all.

Tuskegee's mission has always been to provide service to people in addition to education. The University stresses the need to educate the whole person, that is, the hand and the heart as well as the mind. Tuskegee enrolls more than 3,000 students and employs approximately 900 faculty and support personnel. Physical facilities include more than 5,000 acres of forestry and a campus consisting of more than 100 major buildings and structures. Total land, forestry, and facilities are valued in excess of $500 million. The campus has also been declared a historical site by the United States Department of the Interior.

Historically, Tuskegee University School of Veterinary Medicine (TUCVM) was established in 1945 for the training of African-Americans during a time when few had the opportunity to study veterinary medicine because of segregation and other racial impediments.

The Tuskegee University College of Veterinary Medicine (TUCVM) was established in 1945 and is the only veterinary medical professional program located on the campus of a Historically Black College or University (HBCU) in the United States. The TUCVM has educated over 70 percent of the Nation's African American veterinarians, and is recognized as the most diverse of all 30 Schools/Colleges of Veterinary Medicine in the U.S. The primary mission of the TUCVM is to provide an environment that nurtures and promotes a spirit of active, independent and self-directed learning, teaching, research and service in veterinary medicine and related disciplines.

Also, TUCVM's graduates have excelled in private clinical practice, public practice such the government, military, and in corporations such as the pharmaceutical industry. They hold key leadership positions in the government, military, academia, and in the international arena.

APPLICATION INFORMATION

Supplemental application fee: TUCVM requires a $100.00 supplemental fee. Send supplemental application fee directly to: Office of Veterinary Admissions, Tuskegee University College Veterinary Medicine, Tuskegee, Al 36088.

PREREQUISITES FOR ADMISSION

Courses and Requirements in Semester Hours

I. English or Written Composition	6
II. Mathematics	6
III. Social Sciences / Humanities	6
IV. Liberal Arts	6
	24
V. Biological & Physical Sciences	
Advance Biology (300 Level or Above)**	9
Biochemistry w/Lab	4
Advance Biology Electives	8
Organic Chemistry w/Lab	4
Physics w/Lab	8
	33
VI. Medical Terminology (Effective 2018)	1
VII. Animal Science	
Introduction to Animal Science	3
Animal Nutrition	3
	6
Total Semester Hours (Effective 2018)	**64**

** Advanced biology courses, e.g., anatomy, physiology, ecology, immunology, zoology, microbiology, genetics, toxicology, and histology

All required science courses (Advance biology, biochemistry, chemistry, physics) must have been completed within six (6) calendar years of the time of admission.

For specific application information (availability, deadlines, fees, and VMCAS), please refer to the contact information listed above, or visit the online application process at: http://aavmc.org/Students-Applicants-and-Advisors/Veterinary-Medical-College-Application-Service.aspx.

Residency implications: applications are accepted with special consideration given to Alabama residents and those who have residency in the following contract states, Kentucky, and South Carolina.

Number of resident seats and non-resident seats: none - TUCVM maintains "open access" and selection for seats.

International applications will be considered for admissions into TUCVM

PREREQUISITES FOR ADMISSION

The Tuskegee University College of Veterinary Medicine's professional curriculum is a rigorous four-year program. Therefore applicant's final grade for each required course must be a "C" or better. Students are required to take the General Aptitude portion of the Graduate Record Examination (GRE). Additionally, there is a mandatory interview with the TUCVM Admissions Committee before acceptance into the school is granted.

GPA: the minimum cumulative and science GPA requirement is 2.7 on a 4.00 scale.

Course completion deadline: must be completed by the end of May of the application year.

Effective 2018: Tuskegee will require successful completion of *all* prerequisites prior to application to the College of Veterinary Medicine.

Tuskegee will require a minimum of 200 clinical contact hours with a licensed veterinarian.

Standardized examinations of the application year: Graduate Record Examination (GRE) of which must be taken within three years of application, is required. Must be completed by September 1. Request GRE Test Scores results by October 1.

SUMMARY OF ADMISSION PROCEDURE

Effective 2017: Students will require a minimum of 100 contact hours with a licensed veterinarian in a clinical setting.

Effective 2018: Students will require a minimum of 200 contact hours with a licensed veterinarian in a clinical setting.

Timetable

VMCAS application deadline: September 15 at 12 Midnight Eastern Time

Date interviews are held: January-February

Date offers of acceptances mailed: March-April

School begins: mid-August

Deferments: one-year deferments are considered on a case-by-case basis.

EVALUATION CRITERIA

The following items are taken into consideration: academic record, academic trends, letters of recommendation, work experience, and test scores.

	% weight
Grades	68
Test scores	8
Animal/veterinary experience	6
Interview	15
References	
Science Professors	2
Veterinarian	1
Essay (Handwritten, see application)	

Number of available seats: Approximately 65-70

EXPENSES FOR THE 2017–2018 ACADEMIC YEAR

Tuition and fees

Tuition: $20,585 per semester

Technology fee: $500.00

I.D. fee: $30.00

Supplemental application fee: $100.00

If admitted, additional fees and expenses are required.

DUAL-DEGREE PROGRAMS

Combined DVM–Graduate Degree Programs are available: PhD in Integrative Biosciences, PhD Interdisciplinary Pathobiology, Master of Science Veterinary Science, Master of Public Health and Master of Science in Public Health.

FOURTH-YEAR PROFILE: JOSEPH MASCIANA

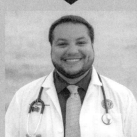

School you are attending
St. George's University; North Carolina State University

What has been your favorite thing about attending veterinary school so far?
The professors. They are the most amazing and the most supportive. I know that if I ever have a question, professional or personal, they will always be there to help guide me. I have made some great connections and am so proud to call my professors my friends and future colleagues.

What advice do you have for prospective veterinary school applicants?
Study hard, but also make time for fun. You want to avoid burnout. I'm guilty of pulling all-nighters every once in a while, but you can't constantly do that. Find at least one thing you like and make a point to do it: hiking, swimming, running, reading, Netflix binge (keep your eye on the time).

What are your short-term / long-term goals?
Short-term is to graduate and pass the NAVLE. Long-term goals are to be accepted into an internship, then residency, and eventually board certify in the American College of Veterinary Emergency and Critical Care.

What extracurricular activities are you involved in during veterinary school?
I was a co-president of Angels in Armor Animal Rescue Fund, which helped un-owned animals in need of emergency or critical medical attention. I was also a facilitator for our Professionalism Attributes Workshops, which help acclimate first-term students to vet school and the island. I was also a tour guide and student counselor in addition to being an active member of several organizations.

What was the biggest challenge you faced during veterinary school?
Finding the "me" time to relax. It was definitely a struggle, but once I got into the rhythm, it was a lot easier to stay on top of my studies and take on additional responsibilities. Also, I got homesick every once in a while, but between Skype, FaceTime, Facebook, and so forth, it was so easy to stay in touch with my loved ones back home.

What advice do you have for other students who are currently in veterinary school?
Figure out the best way you retain information and study in that modality. People study differently, so just make sure your study time is actually valued time.

Why do you want to be a veterinarian?
I want to be able to help families and animals who are having some of the worst moments that they may have in their lives. Knowing that I can advocate for the animal and help all I can is really what I love doing.

What field of veterinary medicine are you interested in pursuing and why?
Small Animal Emergency and Critical Care: Having a patient come into the hospital in very bad shape and watching them walk out tails wagging is what I want to help create more of.

VIRGINIA-MARYLAND
COLLEGE OF VETERINARY MEDICINE

Email Address: dvmadmit@vt.edu
Website: http://www.becomeavet.vetmed.vt.edu

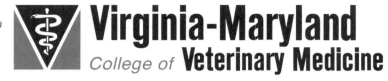

SCHOOL DESCRIPTION

The Virginia-Maryland College of Veterinary Medicine is situated on the campus of Virginia Tech in Blacksburg, Virginia. Blacksburg is located in southwest Virginia between the Blue Ridge and Allegheny Mountains and is a distinct community with a population of about 40,000. Its residents enjoy a wide range of educational, social, recreational, and cultural opportunities. In addition to the main campus in Blacksburg, there are two other campuses, the Equine Medical Center, located in Leesburg, Virginia, and the Gudelsky Center, which is located on the campus of the University of Maryland, College Park.

> Comprehensive four-year curriculum enables students to integrate knowledge, skills, and professional attributes.

Our comprehensive four-year curriculum enables students to integrate their knowledge, skills, and professional attributes within diverse learning environments, all while focusing on the major areas of veterinary medicine. Students will gain proficiency while learning in the large classroom, small group integrative sessions, clinical skills center, and laboratories. After two years of preclinical coursework, students will begin their first clinical experience. The clinical teaching time spans two summer semesters, after which students will immerse themselves in higher level coursework within one of five emphasis areas. At the end of this second teaching time, students will complete their extensive veterinary training within the clinical setting.

APPLICATION INFORMATION

For specific application information (availability, deadlines, fees, and VMCAS participation), please refer to our website at: http://www.becomeavet.vetmed.vt.edu

Residency implications: 50 positions are reserved for Virginia residents, and 30 positions for Maryland residents. Up to 40 additional positions may be filled by nonresidents, 6 of those reserved for WV residents.

SUMMARY OF ADMISSION PROCEDURES

Timetable

Supplemental application deadline: September 15, 2017 (The supplemental application can be accessed at: www.becomeavet.vetmed.vt.edu/howto/steps_to_apply, and will open on June 1, 2016.)

Date interviews are held: January 14 and 15, 2017

Date acceptances mailed: February 14, 2017

School begins: August 21, 2017

Deposit (to hold place in class): $400 for residents and non-residents

Deferments: case-by-case basis if a candidate has extenuating circumstances beyond his or her control

EVALUATION CRITERIA

The admission procedure is comprised of an initial screening of applicants, review of the application portfolios, and interviews of selected applicants.

PREREQUISITES FOR ADMISSION		
Course Description	**Number of Hours/Credits**	**Necessity**
General Biology	8	Required
Organic Chemistry	6	Required
General or Introductory Physics	8	Required
Biochemistry	3	Required
Humanities/Social Sciences	6	Required
Math: algebra, geometry, trigonometry, calculus, or statistics	6	Required
English (3 semester hours must be English composition or a writing-intensive designated course)	6	Required

Pre-Interview Evaluation

60%: Academics: cumulative GPA, required science GPA, last 45 semester hour GPA, GRE aptitude

40%: Non-Academics: related animal experience, veterinary experience; research, industrial, and biomedical experiences; references; and overall application portfolio review

Interviews

Top candidates ranked on the above criteria will be invited to participate in the Multi mini Interview process. Admissions will be based on interview results.

ENTRANCE REQUIREMENTS

Students must earn a "C-" or better in all required courses.

Science courses taken 7 or more years ago may be repeated or substituted with higher-level courses with the written consent of the admissions committee.

Advanced placement credit for 1 semester of English will be accepted if the additional required hours are composition or technical writing and are taken at a college or university.

Advanced placement credit or credit by examination for preveterinary course requirements will be accepted. Those credits must appear on the applicant's college transcript. Advanced placement credits will not be calculated in grade point averages and no grade assigned. No course substitutions will be allowed for AP credit or credit by examination.

Course completion deadline: required courses must be completed by the end of the spring term of the year in which matriculation occurs.

Standardized examinations: GRE not required.

Letters of recommendation: Letters of recommendations are not required. However, letters of recommendation may be submitted electronically through VMCAS and will be reviewed with the rest of the application.

ADDITIONAL REQUIREMENTS AND CONSIDERATIONS

Maturity and a broad cultural perspective

Evidence of potential, and appreciation of the career opportunities for veterinarians, as indicated by:
1. Clinical veterinary experience (private practice)
2. Animal experience in addition to time spent working with a veterinarian
3. Biomedical/research experience (such as working with veterinarians or other biomedically trained individuals in health care, government, research laboratories, industrial, or corporate settings.)
4. Extramural activities, achievements, honors
5. Communication skills

Is a Bachelor's Degree Required? no

Is this an International School? no

ESTIMATED TUITION

Estimated Tuition Resident: $23,617 per year

Estimated Tuition Non-Resident: $50,753 per year

AVAILABLE SEATS

Virginia Residents: 50

Maryland Residents: 30

West Virginia Contract Seats: 6

Non-Residents: 34

VMCAS Participation: full

Accepts International Students? yes

ADDITIONAL INFORMATION

Application Deadline: 9/15/2017

WASHINGTON STATE UNIVERSITY

Email Address: admissions@vetmed.wsu.edu
Website: www.dvm.vetmed.wsu.edu

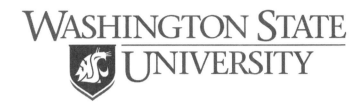

SCHOOL DESCRIPTION

The Washington-Idaho-Montana-Utah (WIMU) Regional Program in veterinary medicine is a partnership between the Washington State University College of Veterinary Medicine, University of Idaho Department of Animal and Veterinary Science, Montana State University, and Utah State University School of Veterinary Medicine. Our program accepts students from all of our contract states and seats are available for non-residents on both the WSU and USU campuses. The WSU College of Veterinary Medicine is also a partner with the Western Interstate Commission of Higher Education (WICHE) program and welcomes WICHE-sponsored students from Arizona, Hawaii, Montana, Nevada, New Mexico, North Dakota, and Wyoming.

> The Washington-Idaho-Montana-Utah (WIMU) Regional Program in veterinary medicine is a partnership.

Washington State University

Washington State University is in Pullman, a town in southeastern Washington. Located in the Palouse region of the Inland Northwest, Pullman offers the benefits of small-town living with the cultural richness of bigger city life. The 60,000 people who live in the communities of Pullman and neighboring town, Moscow, Idaho, enjoy a lifestyle that combines a beautiful country setting with the benefits of two major universities (University of Idaho is just a few miles away). WSU is also a member of the PAC-12 athletic conference, offering exciting sporting events throughout the year. With a true four-season climate, beautiful rivers, nearby mountains and scenic mountain lakes, it's easy to take advantage of a variety of excellent recreational activities including hiking, mountain biking, skiing, snowboarding, fishing, camping and whitewater rafting.

The WSU College of Veterinary Medicine was founded in 1899 and is one of the longest established colleges of veterinary medicine in the country. Several major buildings house the Departments of Veterinary Clinical Sciences, Integrative Physiology and Neuroscience, Veterinary Microbiology and Pathology, and the School of Molecular Biosciences. The college also includes the Veterinary Teaching Hospital, the Washington Animal Disease Diagnostic Laboratory and the Paul G. Allen School for Global Animal Health.

Hands-on experience at WSU begins on day one with caseloads that provide extensive experience in all areas of interest including small animal, food animal, equine, and exotics. Because WSU clinicians have a wide range of specialty areas, the Veterinary Teaching Hospital sees a large and diverse caseload. Students are encouraged to spend time in the Veterinary Teaching Hospital throughout all four years of study. The DVM program also allows for students to take advantage of numerous off-campus clinical opportunities in all areas of veterinary medicine. There are interactive case opportunities at our satellite locations in Spokane, Washington, and Caldwell, Idaho, our primary care programs in partnership with the Seattle Humane Society and Idaho Humane Society, and our affiliate preceptor clinics scattered throughout the Northwest.

The WSU College of Veterinary Medicine is also a leader of innovative educational programs. Before students even take their first veterinary class, they begin their education with an on-site and off-site retreat designed to promote collaboration and team building.

PREREQUISITES FOR ADMISSION

Course requirements and semester hours

Biology (with lab)	8
Inorganic chemistry (with lab)	8
Organic chemistry (with lab)	4
Physics (with lab)	4
Math (algebra or higher)	3
Genetics	3-4
Biochemistry	3
Statistical methods	3
Arts/Humanities/Social Sciences/History*	21
English composition/Communication*	6
TOTAL	**64**

*General education requirements will be waived if a student has a bachelor's degree.

By the time students enter their second year, they have already studied ethics, service, and leadership in veterinary medicine. In their second and third years, students take classes to learn skills in clinical communication, diagnostic reasoning, and may elect to take courses on how to manage a veterinary practice as a part of the Veterinary Business Management Association Certificate Program. Students at WSU have multiple opportunities to engage in dynamic research programs throughout all four years. Opportunities include the Research Scholars Program, Summer Research Program, Research Elective/Supplemental Core Courses, Northwest Bovine Veterinary Experience Program, and combined DVM/graduate studies.

Utah State University

Utah State University is nationally and internationally recognized for its research in animal and biomedical sciences. USU's School of Veterinary Medicine offers an academically outstanding path to pursue a professional degree in veterinary medicine. Classes are taught by faculty from the Department of Animal, Dairy, and Veterinary Sciences and are held in state-of-the-art teaching facilities on the Logan, Utah campus. With dedicated faculty and up to 30 students per class, students will experience a supportive environment for active learning. Students spend their first two years in Logan and then transfer to Pullman for their remaining two years.

Cache Valley is one of Utah's hidden treasures, and Logan, with its population of just under 50,000 residents, sits at the heart of it. Cache Valley lies 83 miles north of Salt Lake City and is a land of dairy farms, small towns, and friendly people. The majestic mountains provide outstanding all-season outdoor recreation, and there are plenty of historical, musical, and art events, plus numerous dining, lodging, and shopping offerings.

Montana State University

Montana State University is a public university located in Bozeman, Montana. It is the state's land grant university and primary campus in the Montana State University System. MSU is ranked in the top tier of US research institutions by the Carnegie Foundation for the Advancement of Teaching. Montana residents spend their first year in Bozeman and then transfer to Pullman for their remaining three years.

Bozeman is located in the beautiful Gallatin Valley, and is a safe and supportive community offering significant opportunity to combine a fantastic educational experience with the great outdoors. Bozeman has a population close to 42,000 residents, making it the fourth largest city in Montana. The area offers fantastic hiking and backpacking opportunities in the surrounding mountain ranges, and the skiing and fishing is some of the best in the country. Yellowstone National Park is a short drive to the south, offering year round recreational activities.

WIMU and WICHE Program Details

Students applying as Washington residents are competing for up to 55 spots for Washington residents only. Students applying as Idaho residents are competing for up to 11 spots for Idaho residents only. Students accepted from the Washington and Idaho pools complete all four years on the WSU Pullman campus. The joint program between WSU/USU seats up to 20 Utah residents and up to 10 nonresidents to spend their first two years in Logan, Utah. Much of the curriculum is taught by the faculty of USU's Department of Animal, Dairy, and Veterinary Sciences, paralleling the curriculum taught in Pullman. The final two years are completed at the WSU Pullman campus. Students applying as Montana residents are competing for up to 10 spots for Montana residents only as a part of the regional cooperative program. Students selected for this joint program spend their first year in Bozeman, Montana, where classes, which parallel those in Pullman, are taught by experienced health science educators. The final three years are completed at the WSU Pullman campus. There are up to 25 spots available for WICHE-sponsored and nonresident students at the WSU Pullman Campus.

Upon satisfactory completion of our program, the Doctor of Veterinary Medicine (DVM) degree is conferred by the Regents of Washington State University. Although the University of Idaho, Montana State University, and Utah State University are partners in the program, all students receive their DVM degrees from Washington State University.

APPLICATION INFORMATION

All applicants, regardless of residency, must complete the VMCAS application and WSU/WIMU Supplemental Application. Applicants must declare their state of residency on the VMCAS and WSU/WIMU Supplemental Application. By identifying yourself as a Washington resident, Idaho resident, Montana resident, Utah resident, a resident of a WICHE state (Arizona, Hawaii, Montana, Nevada, New Mexico, North Dakota, Wyoming), or as a nonresident, your application will be funneled through the appropriate application pool. It is highly recommended that applicants contact the appropriate state authority for information regarding residency requirements as early in the application process as possible.

For the most current application information (details, availability, deadlines, fees, and VMCAS participation), please refer to www.dvm.vetmed.wsu.edu as well as the contact information listed above.

Residency implications: In general, first preference is given to qualified applicants who are residents of Washington, Idaho, Montana, Utah, and qualified applicants sponsored by WICHE contract states. Second preference is given to qualified nonresident applicants.

At the Pullman site there are up to 55 available seats for Washington residents, up to 11 for Idaho residents, and up to 25 for WICHE-sponsored and nonresident students.

At the Logan site there are up to 20 available seats for Utah residents and up to 10 for nonresident students.

At the Montana site there are up to 10 available seats for Montana residents.

SUMMARY OF ADMISSIONS PROCEDURES

Timetable

VMCAS application deadline: Friday, September 15, 2017 at 12 Midnight Eastern Time

WSU/WIMU Supplemental deadline: Friday, September 22, 2017 by 5 PM Pacific Time (The supplemental application can be accessed at: www.dvm.vetmed.wsu.edu)

Interview dates: November-February

Acceptance letters mailed: November-April

School begins: late August

Deposit (to hold place in class): none required

Deferments: considered on a case-by-case basis

EVALUATION CRITERIA

Applicants are selected based upon ability to successfully complete the program and demonstration of the qualities that make a successful veterinarian. Academic criteria include grades, quality and rigor of academic program and GRE test scores. Non-cognitive factors include animal, veterinary, research, and work experience; honors and awards; community service and extracurricular activities; written essay; and letters of recommendation. Other factors include maturity, integrity, compassion, communication skills, and desire to contribute to society. An interview is required for Washington, Idaho, Montana, and Utah residents, as well as for nonresident applicants. WICHE applicants who are certified as residents of their contract state are ranked for participation in the WICHE program using the same criteria above minus the interview.

2016 ADMISSIONS SUMMARY

	Number of Applicants	Number of New Entrants
Washington	151	51
Idaho	29	12
Montana	20	10
Utah	41	22
WICHE states	160	23
(18 WICHE sponsored)		
Nonresident	887	14
Total	**1,288**	**132**

(92 Pullman / 30 Logan / 10 Bozeman)

EXPENSES FOR THE 2016-2017 ACADEMIC YEAR

Tuition and fees – Pullman Site

Resident (WA, ID, and WICHE supported): $24,350

Nonresident: $55,404

Tuition and fees – Bozeman Site

Resident: $23,345

Tuition and fees – Logan Site

Resident: $22,760

Nonresident with scholarship: $45,814

Nonresident without scholarship: $53,814

ENTRANCE REQUIREMENTS

Required undergraduate GPA: No minimum requirement.

AP credit policy: Must meet Washington State University requirements.

Course completion deadline: Prerequisite courses must be completed before time of matriculation.

Standardized examinations: Graduate Record Examination (GRE) General Test is required. Test scores older than 5 years will not be accepted. Test scores are due by September 15, 2017.

ADDITIONAL REQUIREMENTS AND CONSIDERATIONS

Animal/veterinary/research/work experience

Letters of Recommendation. Both an academic and DVM letter are required. A minimum of three letters and a maximum of six letters will be reviewed by the admissions committee.

Extracurricular and community service activities, honors and awards

Personal Statement

WSU/WIMU Supplemental Application

Is a Bachelor's Degree Required? no

Is this an International School? no

TEST REQUIREMENTS

Standardized examinations: Graduate Record Examination (GRE) General Test is required. Test scores older than 5 years will not be accepted. Test scores are due by September 15, 2017.

VMCAS Participation: full

Accepts International Students? yes

ADDITIONAL INFORMATION

VMCAS Application Deadline: 9/15/2017

WSU/WIMU Application Deadline: 9/22/2017

WESTERN UNIVERSITY OF HEALTH SCIENCES

Email Address: admissions@westernu.edu
Website: http://www.prospective.westernu.edu
/veterinary/requirements-17
Link to Application: http://prospective.westernu
.edu/veterinary/apply-17

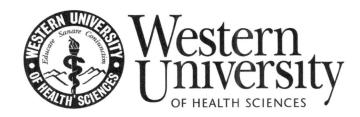

SCHOOL DESCRIPTION

Western University of Health Sciences is an independent, accredited, nonprofit university incorporated in the State of California, dedicated to educating compassionate and competent health professionals who value diversity and a humanistic approach to patient care. The university, located in the San Gabriel Valley of Southern California, about 30 miles east of Los Angeles, grants post baccalaureate professional degrees in nine colleges: the College of Podiatric Medicine, the College of Dental Medicine, the College of Optometry, the Graduate College of Biomedical Sciences, the College of Allied Health Professions, the College of Graduate Nursing, the College of Osteopathic Medicine of the Pacific, the College of Pharmacy, and the College of Veterinary Medicine. The American Veterinary Medical Association Council on Education granted the College of Veterinary Medicine full accreditation status in 2010. Western U's CVM admitted its charter class Fall 2003. The founding principles of the College of Veterinary Medicine include:

> Western University is dedicated to educating compassionate and competent health professionals.

1. Commitment to student-centered, life-long learning. The curriculum is designed to teach students to find and critically evaluate information, to enhance student cooperative learning, and to provide an environment for professional development.

2. Commitment to a Reverence for Life philosophy in teaching veterinary medicine. The College strives to make the educational experience one that enhances moral development of its students and is respectful to all animals and people involved in its programs. Students only practice clinical and surgical skills on live animals when it is medically necessary for that animal.

3. Commitment to excellence of student education through strategic partnerships in the public and private veterinary sectors.

This commitment seeks to maximize the learning experience in veterinary clinical practice and to educate practice-ready veterinarians capable of functioning independently upon graduation. In the 3rd and 4th years of the curriculum students are trained primarily off-campus at state of the art facilities.

APPLICATION INFORMATION

For specific application information (availability, deadlines, fees, and VMCAS participation), please refer to the contact information listed previously.

Residency implications: applicants from all states as well as international applicants will be considered. In-state and out-of-state applicants are given equal consideration.

SUMMARY OF ADMISSION PROCEDURES

Timetable

VMCAS application deadline: Friday, September 15, 2017 at 12 Midnight Eastern Time

Supplemental application deadline: electronically submitted with the prerequisite worksheet RECEIVED on or before Friday, September 15, 2017 at 12 PM PDT

PREREQUISITES FOR ADMISSION

Course Description	Number of Hours/Credits	Necessity
Organic Chemistry with Lab	3	Required
Biochemistry or Physiological Chemistry	3	Required
Upper-Division Biological and Life Sciences with Lab	9	Required
Microbiology	3	Required
Upper-Division Physiology (Animal, Human, or Comparative Only)	3	Required
Genetics	3	Required
General or College Physics with Labs	6	Required
Statistics (General, Introductory, or Bio-)	3	Required
English Composition	6	Required
Humanities/Social Sciences	9	Required

Date interviews are held: November

Date acceptances mailed: mid-December

School begins: August

Deposit (to hold place in class): $500

Deferments: request for deferments will be considered on a case-by-case basis and only after deposit is received.

EVALUATION CRITERIA

Academic achievement

Standardized test performance

Animal experience

Letters of reference

Interview

Other supporting material

Entrance Requirements

Required undergraduate GPA: Applicants must have a minimum overall GPA of 2.75 (undergraduate and graduate) at the time of application to be considered for admission. Prerequisite courses must be completed with a grade of C (or its equivalent) or higher. GPA must be maintained through matriculation into the program.

AP credit policy: must appear on official college transcripts and be equivalent to the appropriate college-level coursework. AP test subject and number of credits must also be specified on the transcript.

Is a Bachelor's Degree Required? no

Is this an International School? no

ESTIMATED TUITION (2016-2017)

Estimated Tuition Resident: $51,810

Estimated Tuition Contract: $0

Estimated Tuition Non-Resident: $51,810

AVAILABLE SEATS

Resident: 47

Contract: 0

Non-Resident: 53

TEST REQUIREMENTS

Standardized examinations: Graduate Record Examination (GRE), general test, or Medical College Admissions Test (MCAT) is required. Test scores must be RECEIVED by the Admissions Office on or before September 15, 2016.

VMCAS Participation: full

Accepts International Students? yes

ADDITIONAL INFORMATION

All courses must be completed at a regionally accredited college or university in the United States. Exceptions will be made on a case-by-case basis.

Coursework completed outside the U.S. (including Canada) must be evaluated by a WesternU approved evaluation service (please visit the requirements page of the website for a listing of approved services).

All required courses must be completed by the end of the spring term of planned matriculation year.

Failure to satisfactorily complete prerequisites with a grade of C or better will result in the loss of a candidate's seat in the class.

One course cannot be used to satisfy more than one prerequisite.

All except two of the science prerequisite courses must be completed by the end of the Fall term immediately prior to the planned year of matriculation at WesternU-CVM.

Application Deadline: 9/15/2017

FOURTH-YEAR PROFILE: JODI RICHARDSON

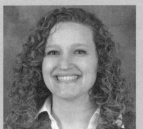

School you are attending
Mississippi State University College of Veterinary Medicine

What has been your favorite thing about attending veterinary school so far?
I feel very fortunate that I have been able to follow my dreams and have fun while doing it. Mississippi State has been so supportive throughout my vet school career in exposing me to numerous areas of veterinary medicine. Additionally, I am grateful to have met classmates and professors who have enriched my daily life and who I know will continue to be lifelong friends.

What advice do you have for prospective veterinary school applicants?
Get some experience doing a lot of different types of veterinary work. When you apply and get accepted, never forget that feeling of when you found out you were accepted to pursue your dream! Be open-minded in vet school—you may end up liking something you never even knew existed.

What are your short-term / long-term goals?
Short-term goals: Graduate. Then go on to pursue an internship in shelter medicine. Long-term goals: I hope to one day enter the Epidemic Intelligence Service with the Centers for Disease Control and Prevention and eventually work for either a non-profit or non-governmental organization improving the lives of people and animals.

What extracurricular activities are you involved in during veterinary school?
Before vet school I played rugby for eight years, and while I don't have the opportunity to still participate in this during vet school, I have found that I love distance running. I have found a group here in Starkville that I run with on the weekends.

What was the biggest challenge you faced during veterinary school?
Being far away from my family has been challenging (I'm originally from Morgantown, West Virginia), but I was lucky enough to make some very close friends early on in vet school, which helped me feel right at home. I also have found it difficult to define exactly what I want to end up doing after vet school because our degree is so diverse and has a lot of interesting aspects.

What advice do you have for other students who are currently in veterinary school?
Work hard every single day, but don't forget to have fun and do what makes you happy. The days in vet school seem long, but four years will go by faster than you think, so remember to be present in each moment and try to soak up as much as you can. One day you're going to be the veterinarian who everyone is looking up to. Throughout the long days, try not to lose sight of why you wanted to join this wonderful profession in the first place.

Why do you want to be a veterinarian?
First and foremost, I love animals. I also love helping people. Veterinary medicine is a unique field where not only do we get to help animals, but we get to help the people attached to those animals, and at the end of the day we can help enhance everyone's life.

What field of veterinary medicine are you interested in pursuing and why?
Before entering vet school I earned my Master's of Public Health. Public health is a field I have continued to stay passionate about throughout vet school, although the role I thought I would play in it has changed. Currently, I am most interested in shelter medicine largely due to the fantastic Shelter Medicine Program we have at Mississippi State that allows us to get hands-on experience in our mobile unit performing high-volume, high-quality spays and neuters. Through shelter medicine I feel that I am making a large impact on the future lives of not only those animals, but also their future owners, and the overpopulation of unwanted pets in our nation.

UNIVERSITY OF WISCONSIN

Email Address: oaa@vetmed.wisc.edu
Website: http://www.vetmed.wisc.edu

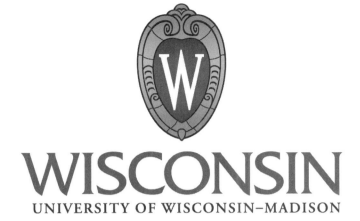

SCHOOL DESCRIPTION

The University of Wisconsin is located in Madison, the state capital, which has a population of about 240,000. Consistently ranked among the nation's "most livable" cities, its hilly terrain, scattered parks, and woodlands saturate the urban setting with a friendly neighborhood atmosphere. Centered on a narrow isthmus among 4 scenic lakes, the city is a recreational paradise. The university sprawls over 900 acres along Lake Mendota and its student population is nearly 45,000. It has rated among the top 10 universities academically since 1910 and is sixth in the country in volume of research activity.

> The University of Wisconsin rated among the top 10 universities academically since 1910.

The School of Veterinary Medicine facility has a modern veterinary medical teaching hospital, modern equipment, and high-quality lab space for teaching and research. The curriculum provides a broad education in veterinary medicine with learning experiences in food animal medicine and other specialty areas. The school pioneered a unique senior rotation in ambulatory service for fourth-year students where they experience the life and work of a veterinarian specializing in large-animal medicine by completing a rotation in one of 24 practices near Madison. The school has an outstanding research program and many faculty members have joint appointments with the College of Agricultural and Life Sciences, the School of Medicine and Public Health, the Wisconsin National Primate Research Center, the McArdle Laboratory for Cancer Research, the National Wildlife Health Labora-

tory, and the North Central Dairy Forage Center. These outside links provide learning, research, and employment opportunities for students.

APPLICATION INFORMATION

To apply for admission, all applicants must complete three (3) online applications: 1) VMCAS, due September 15, 2017 (12:00 Midnight, CDT); 2) Wisconsin's Required Applicant Data Form, due September 18, 2017 (4:00 p.m., EDT) and located at our website: www.vetmed.wisc.edu/radf; and 3) Wisconsin's Supplemental Application. All applicants will be notified by e-mail in November 2017 to complete our electronic supplemental application and to announce its deadline. Interviews are not required as part of the application process.

For specific application information (availability, deadlines, fees, and VMCAS participation), please refer to the contact information listed above.

Residency implications: at least 60 Wisconsin residents will be accepted. Wisconsin has no contractual agreements, but may accept approximately 30 nonresident applicants. Applicants who can claim legal residency or domicile in more than one state should contact the school.

SUMMARY OF ADMISSION PROCEDURES

Timetable

VMCAS application deadline: Friday, September 15, 2017 at 12 Midnight Eastern Time

Interviews: none

Date acceptances mailed: late-February

School begins: late August

PREREQUISITES FOR ADMISSION

Course Description	Number of Hours/Credits	Necessity
Biology or Zoology	4	Required
Genetics or Animal Breeding	3	Required
General Chemistry	8	Required
Organic Chemistry	3	Required
Biochemistry	3	Required
General Physics	6	Required
Statistics	3	Required
English Composition or Journalism	6	Required
Social Science or Humanities	6	Required
Anatomy	3	Recommended
Microbiology	3	Recommended
Physiology	3	Recommended
Cell/Molecular Biology	3	Recommended

Deposit (to hold place in class): none required

Deferments: are considered on an individual basis by the Admissions Committee and may be granted for extenuating circumstances.

EVALUATION CRITERIA

There is a 2-part admission procedure. For the fall 2016 application year, the class was selected based upon the following comparative evaluation:

1. Academic factors, including:
    Undergraduate cumulative GPA
    Required coursework GPA
    Last 30 semester credit GPA
    GRE test scores

2. Non-academic factors, including:
    Animal and veterinary medical experience
    Extracurricular activities and other work experience
    Awards and honors
    Communication skills, maturity and leadership
    Letters of recommendation

ENTRANCE REQUIREMENTS

Required undergraduate GPA: A minimum grade of C (2.0) must be earned in all required courses, including courses completed after application. The mean undergraduate cumulative GPA for the class of 2020 was 3.60 for residents and 3.74 for nonresidents.

AP credit policy: must appear on official college transcripts and be equivalent to the appropriate college-level coursework.

Is a Bachelor's Degree Required? no

Is this an International School? no

ESTIMATED TUITION

Tuition rates are published each year in July; please see our website for details.

2016-2017 Estimated Tuition Resident: $22,762

Estimated Tuition Contract: n/a

2016-2017 Estimated Tuition Non-Resident: $35,906

TEST REQUIREMENTS

Standardized examinations: Graduate Record Examination (GRE), general test, is required. All applicants are required to take or retake the GRE, including the writing assessment. The deadline by which this must be completed is listed on our website. For the most current GRE submission information, please see our website.

A test of English as a foreign language (TOEFL, MELAB, or IELTS scores may be submitted) is required for applicants for whom English is a second language and have not completed an undergraduate degree at an English-speaking college or university. The minimum scores accepted are as follows: internet TOEFL = 100, paper TOEFL = 600, MELAB = 84, IELTS = 7. Please see website for additional information and deadlines.

VMCAS Participation: full

Accepts International Students? yes

Application Deadline: 9/15/2017

INTERNATIONAL
VETERINARY MEDICAL SCHOOLS
AVMA/COE Accredited

ATLANTIC VETERINARY COLLEGE AT THE UNIVERSITY OF PRINCE EDWARD ISLAND

Email Address: registrar@upei.ca

Website: http://www.upei.ca/programsandcourses
/professional-programs/doctor-veterinary-medicine

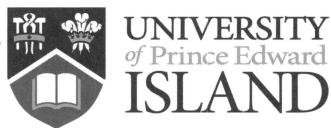

SCHOOL DESCRIPTION

The Atlantic Veterinary College (AVC) opened in 1986 and, since then, has graduated over 1,500 Doctors of Veterinary Medicine. It is fully accredited by the American Veterinary Medical Association and the Canadian Veterinary Medical Association, and is recognized by the Royal College of Veterinary Surgeons (UK).

Located on Canada's eastern seaboard (650 miles northeast of Boston), the Atlantic Veterinary College makes its home in beautiful Charlottetown, Prince Edward Island. With a population of just over 145,000, which jumps to over a million during the summer tourist season, Prince Edward Island is a mixture of rural and urban living, with agriculture, fishing, and tourism the mainstays of its economy. The capital city of Charlottetown (population 35,000) combines a small-town lifestyle with the amenities of larger cities, including dining and theatre. Residents also enjoy outdoor activities, such as golfing, cycling, sailing, and cross-country skiing.

> The Atlantic Veterinary College is a completely integrated teaching, research, and service facility.

The college is a completely integrated teaching, research, and service facility. The four-story complex contains the veterinary teaching hospital, diagnostic services, fish health unit, farm services, postmortem services, animal barns, laboratories, classrooms, information technology services, offices, cafeteria, and study areas.

The AVC Veterinary Teaching Hospital is the most comprehensive veterinary referral hospital in Atlantic Canada and provides care for over 6,000 animals yearly.

Students have the opportunity to work closely with faculty clinicians to manage the care and treatment of dogs, cats, horses, and cattle as well as a variety of other domestic and non-domestic species.

APPLICATION INFORMATION

For specific application information, please visit www.upei.ca/programsandcourses/professional-programs/doctor-veterinary-medicine.

Residency implications: Atlantic Veterinary College contracts with New Brunswick (13), Newfoundland (3), Nova Scotia (16), and the home province P.E.I. (10). International students are admitted on a noncontract basis (26).

SUMMARY OF ADMISSIONS PROCEDURES

Timetable

VMCAS application deadline: Friday, September 15, 2017 at 12 Midnight Eastern Time

Date international interviews are held: November

Date international acceptances mailed: January

School begins: late August

Deposit (to hold place in class): $500.00Can

Deferments: are considered on a case-by-case basis.

EVALUATION CRITERIA

Academic credentials including the GRE are evaluated by the Registrar's Office. Nonacademic ability is evaluated by the admissions committee through an interview process, a psychometric test, and review of the VMCAS application.

% weight
Academic ability 60%
Nonacademic ability 40%

ENTRANCE REQUIREMENTS

Required undergraduate GPA: no minimum stated (under review as stated above); mean cumulative GPA of most recent entering class is 3.70 on a 4.00 scale.

Is a Bachelor's Degree Required? no

Is this an International School? yes

ESTIMATED TUITION

Estimated Tuition Resident: $12,375Can (approx.)

Estimated Tuition Contract: $12,375Can (approx.)

Estimated Tuition Non-Resident: $66,500Can (equivalent to a payment of approx. $25,164US on September 16, 2016, and $25,314US on January 13, 2017)

AVAILABLE SEATS

Resident: 10

Contract: 32

Non-Resident: 26

TEST REQUIREMENTS

Standardized examinations: Graduate Record Examination (GRE). If a student's native language or language of prior education is not English, then the student will be required to submit an acceptable English Proficiency Test score.

VMCAS Participation: full

Accepts International Students? yes

ADDITIONAL INFORMATION

Application Deadline: 9/15/2017

UNIVERSITY OF CALGARY

Email Address: vet.admissions@ucalgary.ca
Website: http://vet.ucalgary.ca/dvmprogram

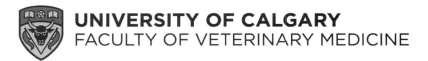

UNIVERSITY OF CALGARY
FACULTY OF VETERINARY MEDICINE

SCHOOL DESCRIPTION

The University of Calgary Faculty of Veterinary Medicine (UCVM) offers a four-year professional degree leading to a Doctor of Veterinary Medicine (DVM). Completion of at least 4 or more semesters of full-time post-secondary instruction at a recognized university or at a college providing university-equivalency in coursework is required prior to application to the DVM program.

> The University of Calgary (UCVM) offers a four-year professional degree leading to a DVM.

APPLICATION INFORMATION

Access to the online application form for the Faculty of Veterinary Medicine can be found on the website (vet.ucalgary.ca/dvmprogram). Applicants must be Alberta residents, as defined by the Province of Alberta. The Alberta Government Guidelines within the Student Financial Assistance Regulations will be used to determine residency status. Details of these requirements can be found on the Alberta Government website at: http://studentaid.alberta.ca/before-you-apply/eligibility/. Proof of Alberta residency will be required with your application.

Completed application forms include the following: complete personal information; a signed statement verifying Alberta residency status and verifying completion of the academic requirements; post-secondary transcripts submitted by the appropriate academic institution; a statement of work experience; and a statement of major extra-curricular activities. Official transcripts should be sent directly from the reporting institution to the UCVM Admissions Office.

English language proficiency must be demonstrated for all applicants for whom English is not their first language.

SUMMARY OF ADMISSIONS PROCEDURES

The Faculty of Veterinary Medicine accepts 30-34 DVM students per year. The Admissions Committee recommends students for admission to the program on the basis of academic and non-academic factors. Students are assessed academically on performance in their last four full undergraduate terms and in ten required courses. Selected applicants are invited for an interview where non-academic factors are assessed. On interview day, applicants are required to complete an on-site essay and participate in a series of interviews and other activities. Applicants must attend interview day at their own expense. There is no entrance exam or requirement to complete the MCAT or GRE exams.

Consistent with UCVM's mandate, preference will be given to applicants who demonstrate the attributes for successful careers in veterinary practice that support rural development and sustainability, and for careers related to our areas of emphasis. While no specific animal or veterinary-related experience is required, such experience is an asset. Understanding of the veterinary profession and animal industries relevant to the applicant's career interests is expected. This can be obtained through practical experience or through other means.

Applicants will be notified of the Admissions Committee's decision in June.

ENTRANCE REQUIREMENTS

All successful applicants are required to forward $500.00 deposit within 15 working days of notification of admission. Failure to do so may result in the position being assigned to another applicant. Such deposits will be applied to the first year's fees. An applicant who accepts a position but later rescinds his or her acceptance will forfeit the entire $500.00 deposit. Successful applicants are required to have or receive immunization for tetanus and rabies following admission.

Is a Bachelor's Degree Required? no

Is this an International School? no

ESTIMATED TUITION

Estimated Tuition Resident: ~$10,860.00 CDN

Estimated Tuition Contract: n/a

Estimated Tuition Non-Resident: n/a

VMCAS Participation: no

Accepts International Students? no

PRE-VET PROFILE: KATHRYN NILSSON

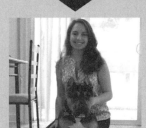

Current School Name
North Carolina State University

What type of veterinary medicine are you interested in pursuing, and why?
I am interested in large animal medicine (both food animals and equine), specifically in reproduction and behavior. I am currently unsure of how to combine the two areas, but I hope veterinary school will be able to shed some light on how to combine and pursue my interests. Although I enjoy dogs and cats, large animals have always been what I am excited to learn about and work with. Theriogenology is fascinating to me, and behavior has been an acquired interest since I started fostering dogs. The breeding/foaling and performance horse management classes offered at North Carolina State University were a great way for me to learn about reproduction and behavior in horses.

What is/was your major during undergraduate school?
I am currently double majoring in animal science with a concentration in veterinary bioscience and zoology. I also have a minor in Spanish.

What are your short-term and long-term goals?
My goals currently are to complete my undergraduate degrees and attend veterinary school. After veterinary school, I hope to do a residency in theriogenology and/or behavior. With a residency under my belt, I aim to work in (or own one day) a large animal practice and participate in as much reproductive medicine as possible.

What are you doing as an applicant/pre-vet to prepare for veterinary school?
From speaking with faculty and current veterinary students, I have seen that studying is a major portion of life in veterinary school. In preparation for this, I am working on figuring out which study method is most successful for me and how I will learn and retain information best.

What extracurricular activities are you involved in currently?
I currently foster pit bulls for the county animal shelter. Most of my time not spent in class, at work, or studying is spent with my dog and my current foster dog(s). Since January 2015, I have welcomed 14 pit bulls into my home and all 14 are now in fantastic homes. In addition, I am active in both Pre-Veterinary Club and Zoology Club.

How old were you when you first became interested in being a veterinarian?
I wouldn't say that I have a specific age at which I knew I wanted to become a veterinarian, but if I had to guess it was in my early teens. My interest was solidified after having my first job at a large animal veterinarian during my first year of college.

Please describe your various experiences in preparation for applying to veterinary school.
Throughout college, my main goal was to get a variety of experiences. I worked in both large and small animal clinics. I also volunteered with NCSU CVM "Turtle Team" my freshman year by helping take care of injured turtles. One summer I completed a two-week large animal study abroad in Belize. Another summer I worked with a North Carolina State University professor and did plant pathology research. In addition to research and veterinarian experiences, I TAed for two animal science classes and was a VetPAC (NCSU's Pre-Vet mentoring/resource office) intern.

What characteristics are you looking for in a veterinary school?
I am mainly interested in veterinary schools with good large animal programs, as well as good theriogenology and behavior programs. Price and location are also important factors.

What advice do you have for other pre-veterinary students?
My biggest piece of advice to pre-veterinary students is to not be intimidated by the process of getting in to veterinary school. It *is* doable. Know what you need to do from the start and steadily complete everything you need to get done. Don't burn yourself out by trying to do everything at once or taking on too much at a time.

UNIVERSITY COLLEGE DUBLIN

Email: vetprogrammes@ucd.ie
Website: www.ucd.ie/vetmed
Phone: +353 1 7166100

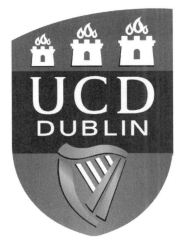

SCHOOL DESCRIPTION

UCD School of Veterinary Medicine is the sole provider of a veterinary medicine degree programme on the island of Ireland, and is one of only five European veterinary schools that are accredited by the American Veterinary Medical Association.

Students of the veterinary medicine programme benefit from the outstanding facilities of the purpose-designed UCD Veterinary Sciences Centre and UCD Veterinary Hospital on the main university campus at Belfield, Dublin (commissioned in 2002). Located on a 132 Ha site 5km south of Dublin's City Centre, UCD is Ireland's largest university with over 23,000 students. This is complemented by Lyons Estate Farm where students have practical classes at all stages of the curriculum.

> The programme is designed to educate you to the best international standards in veterinary medicine.

As the gateway to Europe, Ireland has been renowned for learning and creativity for centuries. Our English-speaking, well-educated population has drawn global companies like Google, Facebook, Intel and HP, who now collaborate with us and employ our graduates.

With its unique blend of urban chic, lush parkland, sweeping coastline, fabulous shopping and excellent cultural experiences, Dublin is without a doubt one of the most energised capital cities in Europe.

UCD is a diverse, international campus. Our student population comprises of more than 50 nationalities, and international students now account for one-third of the total undergraduate student cohort. This diversity is one of the defining features of life at UCD, and one that enriches the student experience by provision of a truly international campus. Your experience as a vet student at UCD will guarantee life-long friendships. You can find further information on attending UCD as an international student at http://www.ucd.ie/international.

Programme/Syllabus

Our veterinary programme is accredited by the Veterinary Council of Ireland, the American Veterinary Medical Association, and the European Association of Establishments in Veterinary Education. It is designed to educate you to the best international standards in veterinary medicine and to prepare you for entry to any branch of the veterinary profession. Veterinary medicine is concerned with the promotion of the health and welfare of animals of special importance to society. This involves the care for healthy and sick animals, the prevention, recognition, control and treatment of their diseases and the welfare and productivity of livestock. Veterinarians also safeguard human health through prevention and control of diseases transmitted from animals to man, through ensuring the safety of foods of animal origin, and through advancing the science and art of comparative medicine.

Veterinary graduates have a wide spectrum of careers to choose from including private practice (companion animals, food animals, horses, exotics, or a mixture of these), government service (animal health, food safety, public health), research or industry.

US applicants through VMCAS are eligible to apply to enter this programme provided they have the prerequisites as outlined below. Further curricular details are published on our web site, www.ucd.ie/vetmed.

The Graduate-Entry Programme is organised into four stages. In stage 1 of the programme students will build on their knowledge of the basic biological sciences by taking modules designed to demonstrate how this knowledge is applied in the practice of veterinary medicine, and gain a firm grounding in animal welfare, behaviour and handling. A key objective will be to ensure that students have the required knowledge, skills and competences to progress to Stage 2. Starting with stage 2 students will take modules with students of the five year undergraduate veterinary medicine programme. As the programme progresses students will learn clinical skills and study each of the clinical sciences using a "body systems" approach. The final year of the programme consists of clinical rotations in the UCD teaching hospital where students have the opportunity to work alongside experienced and specialist staff clinicians, and participate in patient care and client communication. Each student has a personalized timetable ensuring that they participate in rotations in Large and Small Animal Surgery, Diagnostic Imaging, Anesthesiology, Small Animal Medicine, Emergency Medicine, Farm Animal Clinical Studies including Herd Health, Diagnostic and Clinical Pathology, as well as a rotation in shelter medicine. Throughout the programme students are required to participate in extra-mural studies. In the early years, this consists of gaining experience in the handling and management of farm and companion animals, and in later years, of working with veterinarians in practice (clinical extra-mural experience).

APPLICATION INFORMATION

UCD is participating in the VMCAS application system. A supplemental application through the UCD online application system is required.

Fees for Non-European students for entry in 2017 are as follows:

4 year Graduate Entry programme: €36,300*

5 year MVB programme: €30,700*

For further information on entry to the Republic of Ireland, please refer to www.educationireland.com.

SUMMARY OF ADMISSION PROCEDURE

Timetable

VMCAS application deadline: Friday, September 15, 2017 at 12 Midnight Eastern Time

Interviews: January/February (held in the US)

Date acceptances mailed: early April

Deposit (to hold place in class): €2,000, required by early March

Deferments: Not applicable

EVALUATION CRITERIA INCLUDE

Academic performance (a minimum GPA of 3.2 is required)

References/evaluations (minimum 2 required-one from academic science source and one from a veterinary surgeon)

1 page personal statement

Record of Animal and Veterinary Experience

Interview

2015-2016 ADMISSIONS SUMMARY (FOR ENTRY IN 2016)

Resident: 95

Non-Resident: 35

ADMISSION PROCESS

US and Canadian residents must apply to UCD through VMCAS and a supplemental application form which is available at www.ucd.ie/vetmed.

Completed applications are reviewed by our admissions team. Successful applicants will receive their offers from December onwards. Classes begin in early September with compulsory orientation taking place prior to the start of classes.

* For up-to-date information on fees and all further information regarding admission to the University College Dublin, please visit our web site www.ucd.ie.

UNIVERSITY OF EDINBURGH

Email Address: vetug@ed.ac.uk
Website: www.ed.ac.uk/vet

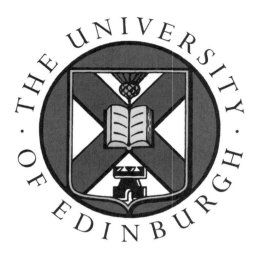

SCHOOL DESCRIPTION

The Royal (Dick) School of Veterinary Studies was founded by William Dick in 1823, and sits within the College of Medicine and Veterinary Medicine at the University of Edinburgh. The School is a recognized world leader in veterinary education, research and clinical practice. The BVM&S degree is accredited by the Royal College of Veterinary Surgeons (RCVS), the American Veterinary Medical Association (AVMA), and the European Association of Establishments for Veterinary Education (EAEVE), allowing our graduates to practice veterinary medicine throughout the United Kingdom, North America, Europe, Australasia and beyond.

> The School is a recognized world leader in veterinary education, research and clinical practice.

Veterinary Medicine at Edinburgh mixes the best of tradition with award winning, progressive teaching. Clinical and professional skills are taught from the earliest stages. Our approach is to ensure optimum integration of the core subjects throughout the curriculum. While many of our graduates enter and remain within the veterinary profession, many others find that training at Edinburgh enables them to succeed in a wide range of careers in research, government, private enterprise and academia.

The Easter Bush campus houses the Royal (Dick) School of Veterinary Studies which incorporates The Roslin Institute, Jeanne Marchig International Centre for Animal Welfare Education and the Veterinary Oncology and Imaging Centre. The Roslin Institute (now the research arm of the Veterinary School) is an animal sciences research institute, which won international fame in 1996, when Ian Wilmut, Keith Campbell and their colleagues created Dolly the sheep, the first mammal to be cloned from an adult cell.

Within the University of Edinburgh, there are over 260 student societies – more than any other university in the UK – covering everything from juggling to horse riding to volunteering, which can cater to your interests. Our sports, music and drama facilities are ranked among the best in the UK.

Edinburgh, the inspiring capital of Scotland, is an historic, cosmopolitan and cultured city, which offers a unique living and learning experience. One of the most vibrant cities in Europe, the city of Edinburgh is regularly voted as one of the most desirable places to live in the world and has been rated the "friendliest city in the UK." This cosmopolitan, safe and welcoming atmosphere encourages all students to feel at home very quickly. With a population of around 500,000, Edinburgh is a compact city, which is easy to travel around on foot or by the efficient public transport network. Edinburgh International Airport has an extensive range of national and international services with direct flights to most major cities in Europe and to a number of major cities worldwide. Many students also take the opportunity to travel around Europe during vacation periods, or even for the weekend, as there are many cheap flight options available from Edinburgh.

For more information on our Veterinary Medicine and Surgery degree programs, refer to the following link: www.ed.ac.uk/schools-departments/vet/studying/bvms-degree.

APPLICATION INFORMATION

For specific application information on availability, key deadlines, fees, VMCAS participation and more, refer to the following link www.ed.ac.uk/schools-departments/vet/studying/bvms-degree alternatively feel free to contact us directly by email at vetug@ed.ac.uk.

Residency implications: For full details and further information on entry to the UK, please refer to https://www.gov.uk/government/organisations/uk-visas-and-immigration. Please note that students must be able to ensure adequate financial support for the duration of their course.

SUMMARY OF ADMISSIONS PROCEDURES

Timetable

VMCAS application deadline: Friday, September 15, 2017 at 12 Midnight Eastern Time

GRE scores deadline: October 1, 2017 at 12 Midnight Eastern Time

Interviews: early to mid-February (held in the U.S.)

Date acceptances mailed: early April at the latest

School begins: early August (4-year Graduate Entry Program), early September (5-year program)

Deposit (to hold place in class): £1,500, required by early May

Deferments: Not applicable. Candidates are not required to submit a supplemental application.

Full details of Edinburgh's application calendar is available here: http://www.ed.ac.uk/schools-departments/vet/studying/overview

EVALUATION CRITERIA

Academic performance

GRE scores

Animal/veterinary experience

Personal statement

Motivation

References/Evaluations (minimum 2 required—one from academic science source and one from a veterinary surgeon)

Interview

ENTRANCE REQUIREMENTS

Graduate Entry (Undergraduate degree-holders or in senior year of degree)

Candidates with a degree (or in their senior year) in an appropriate Biological or Animal Science degree may be considered for the 4-year BVM&S program (Graduate Entry Program). All applicants are required to have completed the required prerequisite courses for the program. US applicants should have an overall minimum grade point average of 3.4 (4 point scale), with greater than 3.0 in science courses. The School also welcomes applications from candidates with an alternative degree who have also completed the required prerequisites. Candidates with a non-science degree would normally be considered for the 5-year BVM&S program. However, if candidates have the specified prerequisites, they may be considered for the 4-year program.

Pre-Vet

Candidates with two years of a pre-vet will be considered for the 5-year BVM&S program. An overall GPA of 3.4 (4 point scale) is expected. All applicants are required to have completed the required prerequisite courses for the program.

Further information about Edinburgh's prerequisites for the BVM&S program is available here: http://www.ed.ac.uk/schools-departments/vet/studying/bvms-degree

Is a Bachelor's Degree Required? yes (4-year GEP), no (5-year)

Is this an International School? yes

ESTIMATED TUITION

Estimated Tuition Non-Resident: £30,200 per annum, fixed for the duration of the program

AVAILABLE SEATS

Resident: 72

Non-Resident: 98

TEST REQUIREMENTS

Standardized examinations: Graduate Record Examination (GRE) general test is required. The scores must be received by October 1 for 2018 entry. Applicants should ensure they take the GRE early enough for scores to be received before the deadline.

Note that the following tests are NOT required for candidates applying to the BVM&S programs at the University of Edinburgh:

- BioMedical Admissions Test (BMAT)
- UK Clinical Aptitude Test (UKCAT)
- Medical College Admission Test (MCAT)
- Veterinary College Admission Test (VCAT)

VMCAS Participation: partial

Accepts International Students? yes

ADDITIONAL INFORMATION

For up-to-date information on fees and all further information regarding admission to the School, please visit our website http://www.ed.ac.uk/schools -departments/vet

UNIVERSITY OF GLASGOW

Email Address: vet-sch-admissions@glasgow.ac.uk
Website: http://www.gla.ac.uk/schools/vet

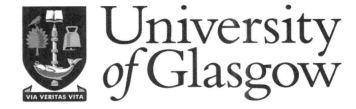

SCHOOL DESCRIPTION

The School of Veterinary Medicine is located on the 80 hectare Garscube campus at the Northwest boundary of the city, four miles from the University's Gilmorehill campus. The School was founded in 1862 and gained independent Faculty status in 1969. In 2010, the Faculty translated from the "Faculty of Veterinary Medicine" to the "School of Veterinary Medicine" within the College of Medical, Veterinary and Life Sciences. The School has a 190 hectare commercial farm and research centre at Cochno, 15 minutes from the Garscube campus (5 miles north).

> The BVMS programme is based on integration of clinical and science subject areas and has a spiral course structure.

The city of Glasgow has a population of around 600,000 and is Scotland's largest city. One of Europe's liveliest places with a varied and colorful cultural and social life, it can cater to every taste. Situated on the River Clyde, Glasgow has excellent road and rail links to the rest of the UK and air services to a wide range of destinations, both home and overseas.

Wherever you come from, you can be sure of building friendships that last a lifetime at Glasgow. According to travel guide Lonely Planet, Glasgow is one of the world's top ten cities.

The School has approximately 200 staff (academic, research, and support) with an additional 65 postgraduate research students, 30 postgraduate clinical scholars, and 600 undergraduate students.

The school is pre-eminent in teaching, research, and clinical provision, and attracts students, researchers, and clinicians from around the world. Our internationally accredited school provides an expert referral centre via the Small Animal Hospital, the Weipers Centre for Equine Welfare, and the Scottish Centre for Production Animal Health & Welfare for animal owners and referring practitioners throughout the UK.

Following the first ever international UK accreditation visit to be undertaken conjointly between the American Veterinary Medical Association (AVMA) Council on Education, the Royal College of Veterinary Surgeons (RCVS), the European Association of Establishments for Veterinary Education (EAEVE), and the Australasian Veterinary Boards Council (AVBC) in April 2013, the University of Glasgow's School of Veterinary Medicine has achieved full accreditation for a further period of seven years.

The BVMS programme is based on integration of clinical and science subject areas and has a spiral course structure, meaning that you will revisit topics as you progress through the programme, each time with increasing clinical focus. In conjunction, there is a vertical theme of professional and clinical skills development to help you acquire the personal qualities and skills you will need in professional environments.

The programme is delivered over five years and is divided into three phases. Years 1 and 2, Foundation Phase, Years 3 and 5, Clinical Phase, Year 5, Professional Phase.

In the recent Research Excellence Framework 2014 (REF2014), the Grade Point Average for Glasgow's veterinary and animal health research activity was ranked top amongst the UK veterinary schools, and in 2015,

QS World University Rankings ranked the veterinary school seventh in the world for veterinary medicine.

EXTRAMURAL STUDIES

In common with all veterinary students in the UK, you will be required to undertake an additional 38 weeks of extra-mural studies (EMS) during your vacation time. The first period of 12 weeks is dedicated to gaining further experience of the management and handling of domestic animals. After this initial period is completed, you start the clinical period of 26 weeks, which can be used to gain experience in veterinary professional environments. Satisfactory completion of EMS is a requirement for graduation.

APPLICATION INFORMATION

For specific application information (availability, deadlines, fees, and VMCAS participation), please refer to the contact information listed above.

Residency implications: Due to recent changes in immigration legislation, students from the U.S. (who are planning to come to the UK for more than 6 months) are now required to obtain an entry clearance certificate prior to entering the UK. For further information on entry to the UK, please refer to https://www.gov.uk/tier-4-general -visa. Students must also be able to ensure adequate financial support for the duration of their course.

SUMMARY OF ADMISSIONS PROCEDURES

Timetable

VMCAS application deadline: Friday, September 15, 2017 at 12 Midnight Eastern Time

Date interviews held: January/February (In the US both East and West Coast)

Date acceptances mailed: April

School begins: late September

Deposit (to hold place in class): £1,000

Deferments: in certain circumstances

EVALUATION CRITERIA

Academic performance
Animal/veterinary experience
References
Essay
Interview
Entrance Requirements
Course requirements
    Applicants are expected to have completed at least 2 years Pre-Veterinary or science courses at College or University, with a minimum of one year in Chemistry (including organic chemistry and organic chemistry lab). We would expect high grades in all science subjects. US applicant should have a minimum 3.4 GPA (4 point scale), and to have achieved at 3.0 in Science.

Required undergraduate GPA: 3.40

AP credit policy: not applicable

Course completion deadline: required courses should be completed prior to admission in the fall.

Standardized examinations: none required. GRE results will be considered if submitted.

ADDITIONAL REQUIREMENTS AND CONSIDERATIONS

Animal/veterinary work experience sufficient to indicate motivation, interest, and understanding of the veterinary profession
    Evaluations: minimum 2, one each from an academic science source and a veterinary surgeon.
    There is no supplemental application for the University of Glasgow.

Is a Bachelor's Degree Required? no

Is this an International School? yes

ESTIMATED TUITION

Resident of UK out with Scotland: £9,000/yr

International: £28,500 (fixed at the point of entry). Fees are set in UK Sterling, and there will be a fluctuation in the exchange rate.

AVAILABLE SEATS

Resident: 72

Non-Resident: 60

TEST REQUIREMENTS

Standardized examinations: none required. GRE results will be considered if submitted.

VMCAS Participation: partial

Accepts International Students? yes

ADDITIONAL INFORMATION

For further information, contact the Undergraduate School Admissions Office (vet-sch-admissions@ glasgow.ac.uk)

Application Deadline: 9/15/2017

UNIVERSITY OF GUELPH

Email: vetmed@uoguelph.ca

Website: www.ovc.uoguelph.ca/ recruitment/en /index.asp

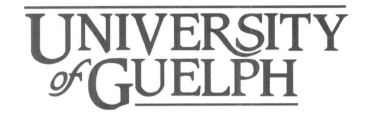

SCHOOL DESCRIPTION

The Ontario Veterinary College (OVC) at the University of Guelph is a world leader in veterinary health care, learning and research. We work at the intersection of animal, human, and ecosystem health.

Founded in 1862, OVC is the oldest veterinary school in Canada and the United States. OVC is located in Ontario, at the University of Guelph, and is a short drive from one of Canada's largest and well-known hubs of activity and culture, Toronto. A drive north takes you to the first of Canada's many popular lakes, known for clear waters and havens of nature.

> The Ontario Veterinary College works at the intersection of animal, human, and ecosystem health.

Academically, OVC is consistently ranked as one of Canada's top universities. In fact, we're renowned worldwide for excellence in teaching, research and service, with graduates of the program practicing veteri-nary medicine, conducting research or working in related industry across the globe.

With faculty and administration sharing like-minded ideas on furthering animal care, research and innovative teaching methodologies, OVC offers a rich and intense learning environment to students. Teaching hospital and facilities specialize in large and small animals, with dedicated intensive and oncology care, mean the potential for hands-on and applied learning are endless.

The University of Guelph, a university consistently ranked the top comprehensive university in Ontario and placed among the top three in Canada by Maclean's Magazine. A national survey of university graduates rated the University of Guelph number one in all but one category, putting it at the top of the list of universities graduates would endorse.

One of five veterinary colleges in Canada, OVC is accredited by the American Veterinary Medical Association, Canadian and American Medical Associations and the Royal College of Veterinary Surgeons of the United Kingdom. OVC grads can be licensed in these countries, giving graduates a spectrum of opportunities.

APPLICATION INFORMATION

Each year, the Ontario Veterinary College (OVC) accepts up to 15 U.S. and international (non-Canadian) students. This year, you could be one of those students!

International applicants must not hold Canadian citizenship (this includes dual citizenship) or Permanent Resident status. Students can apply as early as the summer after their sophomore year provided they have a GPA of 3.2 or above and have done the following prerequisite courses:

- 3 Biology
- Genetics
- Biochemistry
- Statistics
- 2 Humanities/Social Sciences

Course Description	Number of Hours/Credits
3 Biological Sciences (1 with Cell Biology content)	9
Biochemistry	3
Statistics	3
Genetics	3
Humanities/Social Science*	6

*Consider topics such as ethics, logic, critical thinking, determinants of human behaviour and human social interaction.

Applicants who receive an offer of admission should be aware that they must meet federal immigration requirements for entry into Canada as a student.

Non-Canadian applicants who have fulfilled the academic requirements for the Doctor of Veterinary Medicine (DVM) program should apply using the Veterinary Medical College Application Service (VMCAS).

SUMMARY OF ADMISSIONS PROCEDURES

Checklist for non-Canadians applying to the University of Guelph DVM program

Note: if you hold dual Canadian citizenship you MUST apply as a Canadian.

Pre-Application

Complete 2 years of university and the 8 prerequisites within full-time semesters.

Application (September)

Veterinary Medical College Application Service (VMCAS) online application including:

- 3 referee assessments submitted (from 2 veterinarians and 1 professional)

- Background information

- Application fee (to VMCAS)

- The supplemental application form must be submitted separately: http://www.ovc.uoguelph.ca/recruitment/en/applyingtodvm/resources/Prerequisiteform.pdf

- If you are already attending or have attended the University of Guelph please apply using the Application for Internal Transfer/Readmission Form.

Information is gathered through the Academic Background Form (ABF), References, and Transcripts.

November

- Academic Background Form with Course Descriptions (syllabus)
- Supplemental fee

You will be assigned a University of Guelph email account with which you can access your WebAdvisor account for updates on your application status.

November–July

If selected for an interview, you will be contacted by email. Interviews are 45 minutes long with two members of faculty and are usually held at the Ontario Veterinary College in Guelph. Virtual interviews using Skype with a land line are offered for those who cannot visit us in person.

At the end of your on-site interview you will be provided with a tour of the college led by a current DVM student.

Applicants will then be notified by email and letter of the final decision regarding their application.

*Application directly to the University of Guelph is also available and forms can be obtained by emailing vetmed@uoguelph.ca

If you have questions about the application procedure or a current application in progress, please contact:
Kelly Hunter, Admission Services
519-824-4120 Ext. 58711

ENTRANCE REQUIREMENTS

University

Complete at least two years (4 semesters) of full-time studies in college or university. Full-time is usually 12 credit hours at a US school.

All prerequisite courses can be completed in any year of their post-secondary studies. Courses should be completed within an academic program. Courses taken during professional programs or cer-tificate programs are not acceptable.

Students from the US should take a minimum of 12.00 credit hours per semester. Courses must be taken/studied at the same time to ensure an appropriate work load. Field courses or any courses that are pursued over one semester and credited in another semester do not count towards the latter semester's courses for this purpose.

You can study at any accredited college or university and take any major that interests you. You can apply to the DVM program after completing two years of university. If accepted, you do not need to finish your four-year degree program and can simply transfer to the DVM program.

A course that runs the full year will have the credit weight divided equally and half applied to each of the two semesters the course is taken.

Please note that the GPA from your last two full-time semesters, and the average from your 8 prerequisite courses must both be 3.2 on a 4 point scale or higher in order for you to be considered further for entry to the DVM program.

Important Regulations Regarding Acceptable Courses
The specific course requirements listed below must have been completed at the post-secondary level before admission to the Doctor of Veterinary Medicine Program will be considered. Courses do not need to be completed in a designated Pre-Veterinary program.

Courses will not be acceptable if they are repeats of previously passed courses, or if they are taken at the same level or a lower level in a subject area than previously passed courses in the same subject area. This includes courses with significant overlap in content. Students should consider their institution's course sequencing in determining if a course is considered the same level.

The DVM Admissions Committee cannot evaluate Honours, Pass-Fail, and Satisfactory-Unsatisfactory grading systems. Applicants should obtain a numerical or letter grade for all required courses and the grades should be certified by the Registrar of the university attended.

A person's semester/year level is determined by the number of credits that have been completed successfully in his or her degree program plus those that are in progress. Once a person has reached 48 credit hours, he or she is considered a third-year student.

Candidates who hold a non-science bachelor's degree in which they did not take some of the prerequisite courses because they were not part of their program may return to university as part of a non-degree semester(s) to gain the prerequisites. These courses must be assessed by the University of Guelph Admissions Office for content. Applicants with a degree who have a documented commitment, such as work or family responsibility, can present their case to the Admission Committee requesting the option of completing their academic requirements on a part-time basis. This should be done before starting the return to classes. See below for the process.

Failure to comply with the course level rules will result in the exclusion of all coursework from the ineligible semester(s) toward a DVM application.

Course Evaluation Request
If you are not studying at the University of Guelph, you must submit up to two options for the courses that you want to use as prerequisites for approval prior to application.

Requests must include:

- A transcript of university courses completed to date—a photocopy is fine.

- A list of proposed courses for any future semesters you are planning.

- A list of the eight courses to be presented as prerequisite courses and a course description/syllabus for each. You may present one or two choices (no more) for each of the eight. Please be sure to include course codes, titles, and to identify which course is being presented as which prerequisite.

- Your email address and contact information.

Please email course evaluation requests to admdvm@uoguelph.ca and indicate *Course Evaluation Request* with your name in the Subject line.

Appeals Process/Request to Study the Prerequisites During Part-Time Semesters
There are two deadlines to submit an appeal: November 1st and March 1st. Appeals will only be discussed at the OVC Admissions Committee meetings in those months and decisions will apply to the next year's admissions cycle and beyond.

Further instructions can be found on our website: http://www.ovc.uoguelph.ca/recruitment/en/applying todvm/Academicrequirements.asp

Individuals wishing to appeal decisions related to admissions eligibility may submit a letter detailing their individual circumstance and any letters/documentation of support to:

Chair, Admissions Committee,
    Ontario Veterinary College
c/o Kelly Hunter
Admission Services UC L3
University of Guelph
Guelph, ON N1G 2W1
Fax: 519-766-9481
email: admdvm@uoguelph.ca

Please note that appeals may take up to two months to process, and submitting an appeal in no way guarantees a positive response.

NON-ACADEMIC REQUIREMENTS

Veterinary experience
Veterinary experience may be voluntary or paid, but must be done with a supervising veterinarian in placements such as clinical practice, research laboratories, animal shelters, animal rehabilitation facilities, public health settings or another related industry where a veterinarian is employed.

Although there is no minimum required number of hours needed for application, it is strongly advised that applicants log as many hours as possible. Try working with different species, too, such as swine, cows, horses, exotics, dogs, cats, etc. Experience within Canada and the USA is recommended.

Animal experience
Animal experience includes working with livestock, breeding/showing various species, working in a pet store, equestrian activities and any other animal related hobby/experience where a veterinarian is not always present, or does not supervise you. Animal experience does not include pet ownership. Animals are defined as vertebrates for this purpose.

Extracurricular experience
So much of veterinary medicine involves working with people and as part of a service team. Jobs and volunteer activities that hone your communication, interpersonal and organizational skills are important. These experiences do not involve animal contact.

Referee assessments
Three only confidential referee assessments comprised of an evaluative grid and a letter are required for each DVM applicant.

The referees must be qualified to give an unbiased, informed and critical assessment of the applicant. Two of the three referees selected must be veterinarians with whom he or she has obtained veterinary and/or animal experience. There is a strong preference for veterinarians from different clinics or workplaces and may include DVMs in such areas as government, industry, and research. The goal of having the veterinary references is to have those within the profession assess whether you are a suitable candidate to join that profession, therefore it is important that the referees understand what is required of veterinarians in a Canadian/US context.

None of your references should be from family members, long standing friends, or your colleagues or colleagues of your family, even if they are veterinarians. These are not considered objective sources. Your referees should be individuals who know you in a supervisory or professional context and are able to assess you objectively. Applications from candidates with referee assessments from family, colleagues or friends will not be considered suitable for further consideration and will not be invited for an interview.

Graduate students (those from masters or doctoral degree programs) may request an additional form to highlight their accomplishments while within their graduate program.

Is a Bachelor's Degree Required? no

Is this an International School? yes

ESTIMATED TUITION

Estimated Tuition Resident: n/a

Estimated Tuition Contract: n/a

Estimated Tuition Non-Resident: $59,543 Canadian Funds per year

AVAILABLE SEATS

Resident: 105

Contract: n/a

Non-Resident (International): 15

TEST REQUIREMENTS

None

VMCAS Participation: full

Accepts International Students? yes

ADDITIONAL INFORMATION

Application Deadline: 9/15/2017

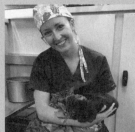

School you are attending
University of Tennessee

What has been your favorite thing about attending veterinary school so far?
My favorite thing about attending veterinary school is the family that I am now part of. University of Tennessee's environment is very close-knit. We rely on each other for support and understand that we are part of the greater veterinary family as well.

What advice do you have for prospective veterinary school applicants?
This is an extremely heavy burden you are about to embark on; do not take it lightly. You will question this decision many times. It is still the best job in the world, if it is right for you. Keep going, study hard, and enjoy the ride.

What are your short-term / long-term goals?
My goals are to begin my career in small animal private practice in Nashville, Tennessee. I want to eventually be a partner in a practice as well.

What extracurricular activities are you involved in during veterinary school?
Intramural sports were always happening through main campus; it was great to go get some exercise and laugh with/at your classmates playing sports against 18-year-olds. Being involved in SCAVMA and class executive board was important to me as I felt I could contribute to the school and better the experience.

What was the biggest challenge you faced during veterinary school?
The amount and depth of material is daunting and very difficult. Moving to a new place and the change that happens in your personal life during veterinary school is also difficult. You grow immensely as a person in a short period of time.

What advice do you have for other students who are currently in veterinary school?
Keep your head up! Clinics is the best part. You learn much much more than you ever thought you could and it all comes together. You are smart, we know that, so don't be afraid to ask questions. Soak up as much information as you can from your clinicians while you have them; soon you'll be on your own. And always enjoy the moment, find humor, and stay positive.

Why do you want to be a veterinarian?
I love the human-animal bond and forming client relationships. Helping people to help their animals is very fulfilling. By using my medical knowledge and scientific curiosity, I can help families to provide happy, healthy lives for their animals.

What field of veterinary medicine are you interested in pursuing and why?
I love small animal private practice; the client relationship is very important to me, and this is what attracts me to practice. Being the family veterinarian and seeing an animal throughout their lifetime, getting to know owners, and also being there during difficult times by lending a kind ear along with medical knowledge are my interests.

MASSEY UNIVERSITY

Email Address: vetschool@massey.ac.nz
Website: www.massey.ac.nz/vetschool

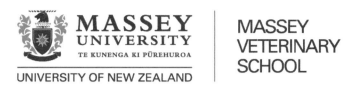

WHY MASSEY UNIVERSITY?

The Massey University veterinary program was the first veterinary program to gain AVMA accreditation in the southern hemisphere. Our program is also fully accredited by the Australasian Veterinary Board Council (AVBC), the Royal College of Veterinary Surgeons (RCVS) and is recognised through reciprocity by the South African Veterinary Association (SAVA). This means you could work as a veterinarian not only in the USA and Canada, but also New Zealand, Australia, the United Kingdom, and many other countries.

> The Massey University veterinary school staff are collegial, motivated, highly qualified individuals.

The Massey University veterinary program has an international reputation for providing an excellent veterinary education with a strong science background, a broad knowledge of companion, equine, and production animal health, and a focus on independent thinking and problem-solving skills. So you can be sure that as a Massey graduate you'll be well prepared for your veterinary career. In fact, in the 2016 QS rankings of veterinary programs internationally, we were ranked the number four program in the world by employers. The QS ranking is currently the only ranking system of veterinary programs around the world (including North America).

JOINING THE MASSEY VETERINARY PROGRAM

We accept up to 24 international students annually, with a total class size of 124. Our veterinary program is 5 years (10 semesters) in length, split into a "pre-selection" phase (one semester—beginning in February annually), and the "professional" phase (the remaining 9 semesters—4.5 years). In the pre-selection phase students compete for entry into the professional phase.

As an international student, you could join our program in one of two ways depending upon your academic background.

Professional phase entry for international students (Group 2)
Group 2 students compete for entry directly into the professional phase on the basis of their academic performance overseas. You need to have completed at least two years full-time or equivalent of an appropriate undergraduate degree. Students selected via this method would start in the professional phase in semester 2 (mid-July). See entrance requirements below for more information.

Pre-selection phase entry for international students (Group 1)
Group 1 international students are those who do not meet all of the eligibility criteria for Group 2, or do but were not selected for a Group 2 position. Group 1 students come to New Zealand and complete the pre-selection phase in order to prove their capability for the professional phase. This is a great option for those who want to get into an AVMA accredited veterinary program who may not be the "traditional applicant".

WHAT IS THE CURRICULUM LIKE?

Throughout years 1-4 you will study core medical sciences (tailored for veterinary students), as well as normal and then abnormal animal structure and function. Then you'll be taught how to "fix" animals, or return them to normal function through clinical studies, medicine, surgery, and health management of companion and agricultural animal species.

A revised curriculum was introduced in 2013 to further increase your learning and understanding by integrating topics within and between years, and introducing problem oriented learning throughout the curriculum. This encourages students to apply the information learned in the various classes to veterinary cases and scenarios designed to develop problem solving and critical thinking. Additionally a greater emphasis has been placed on professional studies, to further enhance your success to further enhance your future career success.

The fifth year is a semi-tracked clinically based year. You would choose a track from the following options: small animal, production animal, equine or mixed animal, or other areas as approved (e.g., wildlife, research). All tracks share a core of 18 weeks of rotations covering multiple species, then depending on which track you choose, you will have a further 7-9 weeks specified. You then have 7-9 weeks where you can choose to do externships (within New Zealand or overseas), or further clinics at Massey University. The semi-tracked, individualized final year curriculum allows you to further explore your area of interest while ensuring wide coverage of the main veterinary species.

During the programme, you will attend lectures, tutorials, practical classes, field trips, clinical sessions and rotations, and undertake farm and veterinary practical work outside of university semester time.

WHERE IS MASSEY UNIVERSITY?

The veterinary school is located in Palmerston North, a student-friendly town of 75,000 in the lower North Island of New Zealand. Palmerston North is a one-hour flight from Auckland, is conveniently close to west coast beaches, and is just under a two-hour drive to the Hawke's Bay wine region, skiing and snowboarding at Mt. Ruapehu and the capital city, Wellington. Nicknamed "student city," Palmerston North offers free bus services for Massey students and has lots of great cafés, restaurants, bars, and outdoor recreational activities.

Renowned for an excellent lifestyle, New Zealand is a great place to study abroad for your AVMA accredited veterinary degree.

APPLICATION INFORMATION

You can find more specific information (deadlines, fees, VMCAS participation, the supplemental application and direct application) on the Massey University veterinary school website.

If you are a US or Canadian resident you can apply to Massey University by either:
1. VMCAS and a supplemental Massey University application or
2. Direct application to Massey University.

All other non-New Zealand residents are to apply directly to Massey University

Residency implications: All non-New Zealand resident students require a student visa, which is easily obtained following an offer of admission into the program. A requirement for a visa is that students must be able to demonstrate financial support for the duration of their course (e.g. Federal Aid loan approval).

SUMMARY OF ADMISSIONS PROCEDURES

Timetable

Group 1

Application deadline: November 1, 2017

Letters of admission to pre-selection (semester 1) sent: Once completed application reviewed.

Pre-selection phase of school begins: Late February 2018 (semester 1)

Acceptances into the professional phase of the veterinary degree program notified: Early July 2018

Professional phase of veterinary program begins: Mid-July 2018 (semester 2)

Group 2

VMCAS application deadline: Friday, September 15, 2017 at 12 Midnight Eastern Time. Online Massey University supplemental application with all supplementary documents to be received by November 1, 2017. Please note, your application will not be processed until you complete your Massey University supplemental application.

Direct applicants: November 1, 2017 (including all supplementary documents)

Date acceptances mailed: from late December 2017

Professional phase of veterinary program begins: Mid-July 2018 (semester 2)

Deposit (to hold Group 2 position): $NZ 1,500.00 (non-refundable)

Deferments: Deferments of Group 1 offers (into the pre-selection phase - semester 1 of the program) are permitted. Offers of a place in semester 2 of the program are for a single year only and as such deferments are not permitted.

EVALUATION CRITERIA

Group 1

The 2018 selection process for Group 1 students is based 50% on academic performance and 50% on non-academic criteria. Please see the website for more detail.

Group 2

Science GPA and GRE: 50%

Non-academic criteria: 50%

This will include an internet based multiple mini interview

ENTRANCE REQUIREMENTS

Course requirements

Group 1: If you are a Group 1 applicant you would come to Massey University to complete a semester (beginning in late February of each year) of full-time science study (4 classes) at Massey University in order to develop a GPA for selection. If you have already taken similar classes to one or more of the four prerequisite classes, you'll be given credit for these and choose alternate science classes to replace them.

Group 2: Competitive Selection directly into the professional phase BVSc Semester 2 (6-10 places available).

To be eligible for Group 2 you would need to have completed at least two full years of full-time, largely science based university education, including classes equivalent to the 4 Massey University veterinary prerequisite classes.

Massey University Class: Usual classes needed for credit

123.101 Chemistry and Living Systems: General chemistry + Organic chemistry

124.111 Physics for Life Sciences: 1 year of physics

162.101 Biology of Cells (molecular) biology +/- First year biology series

199.101 Biology of Animals: Animal biology / vertebrate zoology

Each of the above classes should include laboratories.

Required undergraduate GPA: A minimum science GPA of 3.00 is required to be eligible for selection into the professional phase (Semester 2) of veterinary degree.

Course completion deadline:

Group 1: Not applicable; courses completed in New Zealand.

Group 2: All four of the pre-requisite courses (or their equivalent) should be completed by the end of the fall semester in the year prior to matriculation (e.g., Fall 2017 for matriculation in 2018).

Standardized examinations: Graduate Record Examination (GRE) - General Test, is required for Group 2 applicants only. Test scores should be no older than 5 years immediately preceding the application deadline. Scores must be received by the supplemental application deadline.

ADDITIONAL REQUIREMENTS AND CONSIDERATIONS

All VMCAS applicants must complete the supplemental application for Massey University. Your application will not be processed until you have submitted your online supplemental application.

The supplemental application consists of:
- An online Massey University application form for admission as an international student.

We also require the following but you usually do not need to supply these as they are sourced directly from NAVLE or ETS once you have completed your supplemental application:
- Your GRE score – from ETS.
- Your transcripts – from NAVLE application.
- Verification of your veterinary practical work experience – A letter signed by a veterinarian verifying you have completed a minimum of 10 days (80 hours) work experience at their clinic. ELoR's submitted by veterinarians as part of the VMCAS application can be substituted for the signed letter. Letters of recommendation are not required.

A bachelors degree is not a prerequisite requirement for admission into the veterinary degree.

Is a Bachelor's Degree Required? no

Is this an International School? yes

ESTIMATED TUITION

Estimated Tuition Resident: Subsidized

Estimated Tuition Contract: 0

Estimated Tuition Non-Resident: $NZ 30,185 NZD per semester

AVAILABLE SEATS

Resident: 100

Contract: 0

Non-Resident: 24

TEST REQUIREMENTS

Standardized examinations: Graduate Record Examination (GRE) - General Test is required for Group 2 applicants only. Test scores should be no older than 5 years immediately preceding the application.

VMCAS Participation: partial

Accepts International Students? yes

ADDITIONAL INFORMATION

Please note: The tuition fees are in New Zealand dollars. The actual cost in your currency will depend on the exchange rate at the time of paying tuition fees. The NZD is traditionally lower than the USD and CAD. Historically once conversion rates are accounted for, tuiton fees at Massey University are usually in the third least expensive for out-of-state schools.

Application Deadline: 11/1/2017

VMCAS Deadline: 9/15/2017

UNIVERSITY OF MELBOURNE

Website: www.fvas.unimelb.edu.au

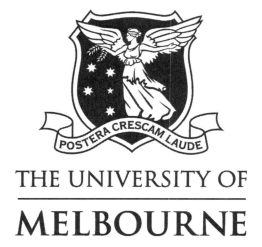

THE UNIVERSITY OF
MELBOURNE

SCHOOL DESCRIPTION

The University of Melbourne has a 150-year history of leadership in research, innovation, teaching and learning. As a University of Melbourne student, you will become part of a dynamic collegial environment with a distinctive research edge. Throughout its history the University of Melbourne has educated some of the world's most eminent scientists and researchers and this tradition continues today. Currently, we are the top ranked university in Australia.

> The University of Melbourne has a 150-year history of leadership in research, innovation, teaching and learning.

The Melbourne Veterinary School's heritage began in 1886 as the first veterinary college in Australia, and celebrated its centenary as a Faculty of the University of Melbourne in 2009. In July 2014, through consolidation of university faculties the new Faculty of Veterinary and Agricultural Sciences was created. The Faculty is now comprised of the School of Agriculture and Food and The Melbourne Veterinary School. Under the leadership of Professor Ted Whittem as the Head of School, our nationally and internationally accredited DVM degree program and our globally respected research and research-training programs are now taught and managed within The Melbourne Veterinary School.

Our DVM veterinary program is delivered across two sites: the city-centre Parkville campus and the regional Werribee campus with our clinical teaching facilities. The veterinary teaching hospital was designed to support top-class veterinary education with facilities which include consulting rooms, modern diagnostic capabilities including endoscopy, CT, MRI, image intensification, scintigraphy, on-site diagnostic pathology laboratories and a 24-hour small animal emergency and critical care unit. Beginning in 2017, the university is transforming both campuses by constructing major additions to the veterinary teaching hospital plus new state-of-the-art teaching facilities.

The veterinary program provides extensive hands-on experience which includes industry integrated practical learning and clinical externship opportunities. Students gain experience in animal handling, care and management by undertaking professional work-experience during and between the academic years. The school has strong programs in specialty disciplines for companion animals, horses, dairy cattle, sheep and beef cattle. The school also has very strong primary care and emergency practices wherein DVM students gain Day-1 readiness. In addition to their broad-based core training, our students select a track in the third year to supplement their learning in a chosen area of interest. As a Melbourne Veterinary School student you will have the opportunity to be involved in extra practical classes and activities with classmates who share your interests. The tracks available are:

1. Production Animals
2. Small Animals
3. Horses
4. Government, industry and conservation health

The DVM degree is accredited by the American Veterinary Medical Association (AVMA), by the Royal College of Veterinary Surgeons (UK), and by the Australasian Veterinary Boards Council Inc. These accreditations reflect the high quality and international standing of the course and permits graduates of the course to work as veterinarians in a wide range of countries including North America. Our success has been achieved by insisting on international excellence. Talented people from all over the world come to visit, study and work at the University of Melbourne. At last count, the University's student community of 44,000 included more than 9,800 international students from over 100 countries.

We invite you to join our tradition and discover why staff and students of the highest calibre are attracted to study at the Melbourne Veterinary School.

COURSE DURATION, ENTRY ROUTES AND STUDENT NUMBERS

The Melbourne Veterinary School offers studies in veterinary education through our professional entry graduate degree: the Doctor of Veterinary Medicine. The four-year degree offers veterinary students the best possible preparation for twenty-first century careers in a rapidly changing and increasingly global workforce. Students can enter the veterinary science program by one of two pathways:

1. As a graduate student by completing a science or agricultural degree at another institution. Students who follow this pathway will enter the four-year graduate entry DVM program.

or at the University of Melbourne.

2. Via the undergraduate pathway by gaining entry to the Bachelor of Science degree at the University of Melbourne and achieving selection at the end of their second year.

NUMBER OF INTERNATIONAL STUDENTS THAT WE ACCEPT

Each year level has a total of 130 students with approximately 50 places reserved for international students.

PREREQUISITES FOR ADMISSION

1. Entrance to the DVM via the Melbourne Bachelor of Science: North American students should refer to the University's international prospectus for up to date details about entrance requirements for the Bachelor of Science by visiting www.course search.unimelb.edu.au.

2. Entrance to the DVM as a graduate: Applicants will require a science or agricultural degree from the University of Melbourne or another institution. Examples of appropriate degrees include Bachelor's degrees with majors in: Agriculture, Animal Science, Biochemistry, Biomedicine, Physiology or Zoology. Prerequisites for entry as a gradu-

ate are at least one semester of study in each of general or cellular biology and biochemistry as part of a science or agricultural degree.

3. Entrance to the DVM as an undergraduate: After completing prerequisite first and second year subjects in the Bachelor of Science, students will be eligible to apply for entry to the Veterinary Bioscience specialisation of the Animal Health and Disease major in third year. Students who successfully complete their studies will have guaranteed entry into the DVM, with credit for one year of study, leaving three years of study in the DVM.

4. There is no standardised test or interview required.

APPLICATION INFORMATION

International applications will be accepted throughout the year. Applications close in late December, for enrolment commencing in February the following year. Applicants are advised to apply as soon as possible to avoid disappointment. Applications will be considered as soon as they are received. We recognise the amount of time required by successful applicants to make arrangements for international travel and study and we attempt to give them as much advance notice as possible. Students apply via the International Admissions Office at the University of Melbourne. They can choose to apply online or apply through one of our overseas representatives. Visit www.futurestudents.unimelb.edu.au/info/international.

TUITION FEES

For information about tuition fees please visit:

- Undergraduate (e.g., Bachelor of Science) http://futurestudents.unimelb.edu.au/admissions/fees/ug-intl
- Graduate (e.g. DVM) http://futurestudents.unimelb.edu.au/admissions/fees/grad-intl

Application fee: AUD$100

Visas: All non-Australian students require a student visa, which is easily obtained following an offer of admission into our program. More information can be viewed on the website: www.services.unimelb.edu.au/international/visas/apply.

Deferments: Please note that successful applicants may not defer commencement of the DVM. Students can reapply for a start year intake when they are able to commence studies, and the application fee will be waived for international students.

NATIONAL AUTONOMOUS UNIVERSITY OF MEXICO (UNAM) COLLEGE OF VETERINARY MEDICINE

Email: fmvyz@galois.dgae.unam.mx
Website: www.fmvz.unam.mx
http://escolar.fmvz.unam.mx

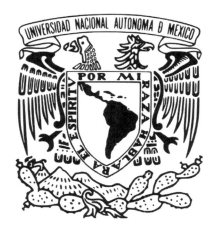

APPLICATION INFORMATION

Undergraduate admission of new students to the National Autonomous University of Mexico (UNAM) is done through the General Administration Scholar Affairs Direction (DGAE).

The applicants to the College of Veterinary Medicine, students are evaluated in terms of their general academic background, with emphasis on Biology, Chemistry, Physics and Mathematics.

> The number of available positions at UNAM is 450, without distinction for Mexican or foreign applicants.

There are two annual applications dates: January and April. Information for specific applications dates can be reviewed at www.escolar.unam.mx (the semester starts in August).

Application forms can be found at the same website. The number of available positions is 450, without distinction for Mexican or foreign applicants.

RESIDENCY IMPLICATIONS

There are no resident implications. All the students have to take the admission test. Recommendation letters are not needed.

PREREQUISITES FOR ADMISSION

Applicants must have at least a high school average grade of 70%.

Minimum of semesters needed in: mathematics, physics, chemistry, and biology

COURSES (Semesters)

Mathematics (4 semesters)

Physics (4 semesters)

Inorganic and organic chemistry (4 semesters)

Principles of biology and general biology (4 semesters)

Social sciences / humanities (6 semesters)

Electives (2 semesters): selected topics on biology, statistics, morphophysiology or physicochemistry

For students from foreign high schools, beside the admission test, they have to submit all necessary official documents to "Dirección General de Incorporación y Revalidación de Estudios (DGIRE) UNAM". Submission instructions can be found at http://www.dgire.unam.mx/contenido/home.htm.

Foreign students whose primary language is not Spanish will have to do a proficiency Spanish language test.

Required undergraduate GPA: It is not necessary

AP credit policy: Is not part of the admission requirements

Course completion deadline: It is based on the application dates, in January and June.

Standardized Examinations: They are not used

Additional requirements and considerations: Foreign students must have a good command of the Spanish language

SUMMARY OF ADMISSION PROCEDURE

Timetable

The next application dates can be checked at www.escolar.unam.mx

Deposit: It is not necessary

Deferments: Considered on an individual basis, and ordinarily granted for personal reasons, illness, lack of economic resources or other situations beyond the control of the students.

Evaluation criteria: Grade of 80% or above in the admission exam.

2015–2016 ADMISSIONS SUMMARY

Number of Applicants	Number of New Entrants
3,285	86 (2.6%)

EXPENSES FOR THE 2012–2013 ACADEMIC YEAR

(subject to change)

Tuition and fees: $2,000 USD per year

Current School Name
North Carolina State University

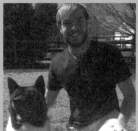

What type of veterinary medicine are you interested in pursuing, and why?
With my diverse experience, I intend to become a veterinarian with a mixed practice for small animals that also takes on wildlife cases. I would like to go into small animal medicine because of my concern for the well-being of people's pets, and I want to be able to treat and heal them. Wildlife medicine interests me because I want to ensure that animals will survive for generations to come.

What is/was your major during undergraduate school?
My major at North Carolina State University is animal science with a concentration in veterinary bioscience and a minor in entomology.

What are your short-term and long-term goals?
My short-term goals are to perform well in veterinary school and to enjoy my time there. I want to gain hands-on work experience with companion animals as well as wildlife. When it comes to long-term goals, I have multiple options I will be deciding from. One option is to buy into a small animal practice and one day become the owner. Another option is I see myself becoming a wildlife veterinarian and traveling across the country to treat numerous different species. I hope through experience to find a way to combine these options.

What are you doing as an applicant/pre-vet to prepare for veterinary school?
I applied to various veterinary colleges in the fall of 2015 and am currently preparing myself for the scheduled interviews that I have in the coming months. Before applying, I researched the veterinary colleges, but during my visits for the interviews I will be focusing on the student atmosphere, diversity, and surrounding area. These demographics will help me decide which is the best fit college for me.

What extracurricular activities are you involved in currently?
While in college, I founded a student club for beekeepers, of which I am the current president. Students with all ranges of knowledge come together, learn, and get hands-on experience working with honey bees. On weekends, I release energy with contra dancing, which is a form of folk dancing that brings people together from all walks of life.

How old were you when you first became interested in being a veterinarian?
Starting at a young age, I had a passion for animals and insects that grew into a curiosity for nature and lead to an interest in actively pursuing science. During my high school International Baccalaureate program, I was required to participate in community and service hours, so I chose to volunteer at a local animal hospital. While assisting the veterinarians and vet-techs with basic animal treatments, my interest in becoming a veterinarian was formalized.

Please describe your various experiences in preparation for applying to veterinary school.
For four summers, I had an internship at a sea turtle hospital where I had hands-on work rescuing and rehabilitating sea turtles. Each morning consisted of feeding, cleaning, medicating, and rehabilitating sea turtles. In the afternoon, we gave tours to tell the stories of each sea turtle as well as educate the public on the dangers that sea turtles faced. Currently, I work at a small animal clinical practice where I experience the daily life of a veterinarian. I get hands-on experience and observe procedures like surgeries, as well as the mix of general practice interfaced with emergency situations.

What characteristics are you looking for in a veterinary school?
When applying to veterinary school, I looked for a school with a curriculum that had small animal as well as wildlife medicine with chances to intern with all different species of animals.

What advice do you have for other pre-veterinary students?
My advice is to diversify your experience; do not just go work with farm animals and companion animals. We live in such a diverse world that you should work with an animal that fascinates you but is outside the typical animals. Pre-vet students can get jobs and internships with animals from around the world. There are possibilities to work with anything ranging from large cats to marine animals to even insects, if that is what you enjoy. There are so many possibilities in the world that you should search outside the ordinary species.

UNIVERSITÉ DE MONTRÉAL

Email: saefmv@medvet.umontreal.ca
Website: www.medvet.umontreal.ca

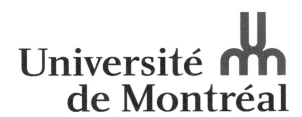

APPLICATION INFORMATION

Applications available: December 1
   Online: 94$CAN

Application deadline: January 15

Residency implications: Canadian citizenship or permanent residency in Canada is required.

A total of 96 students are admitted each year.

> A total of 96 students are admitted each year. All lectures are given in French. Examinations must be written in French.

To be considered for admission, one must: a) meet the above requirements for citizenship, and b) have completed the required studies.

Note: All lectures are given in French. Examinations must be written in French.

The DMV is a 5-year program.

Condition concerning the knowledge of French: To be admissible, the candidate must demonstrate that he/she has acquired the minimal level of proficiency in French as required by the chosen program, as established by the University. To this end, the candidate must either:

- succeed the Épreuve uniforme de langue et littérature française of the Ministry of Education of Quebec or;
- obtain a score of at least 785/990 on the International French exam (Test de français international TFI) http://www.etudes.umontreal.ca/programme/doc_prog/section2.pdf.

Performance Score: This score is obtained by comparing the student's grade in each course with the class average.

Course completion deadline: The applicant must have completed all prerequisites at the time of application.

Additional considerations (in order of importance)
   1. Academic record
   2. Admission test

SUMMARY OF ADMISSION PROCEDURE

Timetable

Application deadline: January 15

Admission test: beginning of january to beginning of April (online test)

Notification of acceptance: end of May, early June

Fall semester begins: end of August

Deposit (to hold place in class): 300$CAN

Evaluation criteria	%
Performance score	60
Admission test	40

ESTIMATED EXPENSES FOR THE 2017–2018 ACADEMIC YEAR

Tuition and fees: 100$CAN per credit for residents of Quebec (approx. 45 per year)

250$CAN per credit for Canadian non-residents of Quebec

PREREQUISITES FOR ADMISSION

DEC (Diplôme d'Etudes Collégiales) including the following courses:

Course requirements

Physics	101, 201, 301–78
Chemistry	101, 201, 202
Biology	301, 401
Mathematics (including calculus)	103, 203

MURDOCH UNIVERSITY

Email Address: international@murdoch.edu.au
Website: http://www.murdoch.edu.au/School-of-Veterinary-and
-Life-Sciences

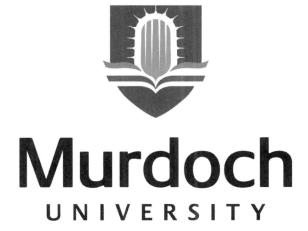

SCHOOL DESCRIPTION

Western Australia is a beautiful part of Australia with a warm sunny climate. It has some of the world's most precious natural phenomena including Ningaloo Reef and the 350-million-year-old Bungle Bungle Range in the north, and the towering Karri forests of the south west. Perth is a modern, safe cosmopolitan city with a relaxed lifestyle that focuses on the outdoors. There are wineries, beaches, bushland, and unique wildlife within easy reach of the city, and a cosmopolitan mix of cafes, restaurants, pubs and thriving nightlife in the city center.

> Veterinary students learn in a true practice atmosphere with the final year of study devoted entirely to clinical exposure.

Murdoch University is a public university based in Perth, with campuses also in Singapore and Dubai. It began operations as the state's second university in 1973, and accepted its first students in 1975. The University is located 15km south of the central business district of Perth, and about 8 kilometers east of the port city of Fremantle. It currently is home to over 22,500 students including approximately 3,000 international students from over 90 countries.

Veterinary students from Murdoch graduate with a double degree (Bachelor of Science [Veterinary Biology] and Doctor of Veterinary Medicine) from a course that takes a total of five years to complete. The course is designed to enable students to acquire the knowledge and skills necessary for the diagnosis, treatment and prevention of disease in pets, farm animals, wildlife and laboratory animals. Veterinary students learn in a practice atmosphere with the final year of study lecture-free and devoted entirely to clinical exposure, including time spent at Perth Zoo.

The Veterinary Biology degree (3 years) encompasses both normal and abnormal aspects of vertebrate structure and function. The first year comprises units which introduce the scientific process, analysis of data and the form and function of the animal body; units in the second year include information on animal development, structure, function and metabolism; and units in the third year cover general aspects of the causes and nature of disease and its control. A further 6 trimesters of study over 2 calendar years leads to a Masters level degree of Doctor of Veterinary Medicine (DVM) which is a registrable veterinary qualification.

Murdoch students have access to excellent facilities, all on the one campus, including a 24-hour emergency clinic, large and small animal practices, an on campus farm and an equine hospital, as well as production animal and equine ambulatory services. The thriving practices have busy caseloads, serviced by many specialist clinicians, so that students can gain extensive experience.

The new BSc/DVM curriculum is designed to keep Murdoch at the forefront of veterinary education. This curriculum allows more time for students to develop areas of special interest through non-core rotations, externships and extramural experience. A Veterinary Professional Life stream is integrated throughout the course to assist students in their transition to future careers in veterinary science and provides a strong focus for developing professional life skills within the veterinary profession.

The veterinary science degree is accredited by the American Veterinary Medical Association (AVMA), the Royal College of Veterinary Surgeons (UK), and the Australian Veterinary Boards Council. Completing your Veterinary Science degree Murdoch saves you years of study, and potentially thousands of dollars; this is because with the correct preparation, the 4 years of veterinary specific tuition can be entered into after only one year of tertiary study in general biological science. Once you have finished your degree at Murdoch, you are eligible to sit your exams with the AVMA just as you would if you completed your studies in North America.

APPLICATION INFORMATION

For specific information (availability, deadlines, fees, and VMCAS participation), please refer to the contact information listed above.

All non-residents require a student visa, which is easily obtained following an offer of admission into the veterinary course. Applicants whose first language is not English must demonstrate competency in the English language, further details can be found at http://www.murdoch.edu.au/Future-students/International-students/Applying-to-Murdoch/English-requirements.

SUMMARY OF ADMISSIONS PROCEDURES

Timetable

There are four application deadlines each year, which are: March 31, June 30, September 30 and November 30.

School begins: mid-February

Some candidates may be eligible to begin in late July.

VMCAS application deadline: not applicable. Students are to apply direct via Murdoch. Application form can be found at http://www.murdoch.edu.au/Future-students/International-students/Applying-to-Murdoch/Application-forms

Deposit to hold a position: $1,000 AUD payable upon acceptance of offer

ENTRANCE REQUIREMENTS

Students who have completed one or more years of tertiary study and who have satisfied the appropriate prerequisites are eligible to apply for entry into second year of the 5-year program. Currently the prerequisites include units in chemistry, statistics and data analysis, introductory animal anatomy and physiology, cell and molecular biology and vertebrae structure and function, plus a unit that explores the basic building blocks for science students and another that introduces the history and philosophy of science and the interconnected nature of scientific disciplines. A unit covering the principles of livestock science in an Australian context is also a prerequisite. This unit incorporates mandatory components that include animal handling competence of the common farm animals and a farm safety course. For students entering at the start of 2nd year a summer version of this unit is available.

Applications are also accepted from school leavers, with high achievers offered a place in the first year at Murdoch with a guaranteed progression into the veterinary specific course, provided they pass all first year units at the first attempt. Other applicants will be formally selected from those who have successfully completed one year or more of tertiary study, including the prerequisite units listed above, or equivalent units (excluding the livestock science unit). Applicants are required to supply with the application form (1) a curriculum vitae (CV) and (2) a typed Personal Statement of up to 500 words to which should be attached documents such references, and which should outline why you wish to become a veterinarian. You should include information such as how you consider your past study and experience to date will assist you to succeed in the veterinary course and in the veterinary profession. If you have any fails/late withdrawals in your post-secondary/tertiary study, you should explain the circumstances for your poor performance and why those circumstances will not apply to your Murdoch studies. You should aim to demonstrate your motivation and preparation for veterinary science

Assessment of the application will be based on the academic standard achieved in all previous tertiary study, the personal statement, and documented evidence of recent veterinary and animal related experience. Applicants who have satisfied the appropriate prerequisites may be offered a place in the second year of the BSc/DVM course. If not, an offer may be made into the first year of the course, with an assured progression into the second year after successful completion of all units in that year at the first attempt.

Deferments: considered on merit

Is a Bachelor's Degree Required? no

Is this an International School? yes

ESTIMATED TUITION

Estimated Tuition Resident: n/a

Estimated Tuition Contract: 0

Estimated Tuition Non-Resident: *A$29,000 progressing to *A$81,000 pa. *Based on 2015 values.

AVAILABLE SEATS

Resident: 0

Contract: 0

Non-Resident: 45

VMCAS Participation: non-VMCAS

Accepts International Students? yes

ADDITIONAL INFORMATION

Application Deadline: 11/20/2017

THE UNIVERSITY OF QUEENSLAND

Email Address: enquire@science.uq.edu.au
Website: veterinary-science.uq.edu.au

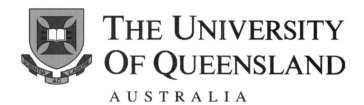

THE UNIVERSITY
OF QUEENSLAND
AUSTRALIA

SCHOOL DESCRIPTION

The veterinary qualification of The University of Queensland (UQ) is accredited with the American Veterinary Medical Association, the Australasian Veterinary Boards Council (Australia and New Zealand), the Royal College of Veterinary Surgeons (United Kingdom), Malaysian Veterinary Council and the South African Veterinary Council.

The School of Veterinary Science's purpose-built facilities are located at UQ's Gatton campus and include Veterinary Teaching Laboratories, the Clinical Studies Centre, and the Veterinary Medical Centre (VMC) with fully equipped Equine and Companion Animal Hospitals, complete with the latest instrumentation for diagnostic imaging and surgical techniques. The VMC has recently commenced an ambulatory service for treatment of production animals on the rural properties surrounding the campus.

> The School has been recognised for a sustained record of excellence in teaching and learning.

The UQ Gatton campus is approximately 40 miles west of Brisbane, the capital city of the state of Queensland in Australia. The campus is easily accessible within one to two hours' drive from the major urban and tourism centres of Brisbane, the Gold Coast and Toowoomba, and has a rural atmosphere with on-campus access to domesticated animals including horses, cattle, pigs, poultry, cats, dogs and wildlife including kangaroos, reptiles and birds.

The School's co-location with the Queensland Animal Science Precinct makes the Gatton campus the most comprehensive animal research and training centre in Australia.

Since its first intake of students in 1936, the UQ School of Veterinary Science has been recognised for a sustained record of excellence in teaching and learning across the veterinary disciplines, and for the quality of its research.

With state-of-the-art facilities, and an ambitious academic recruitment program that has attracted an excellent cohort of staff, the School is at the forefront of veterinary education, supporting UQ's global ranking in the top 100 universities.

The diverse group of academic and clinical staff in the School, including those who have been recognised through nationally accredited awards, have made major contributions to tropical/subtropical animal health and medicine to benefit farm and companion animals, their owners and industry sectors.

The curriculum of the School of Veterinary Sciences is a 10-semester (5-year) program that runs from February to November in the first four years and November to October in the final year. The first year provides core foundational training in biological sciences, with emphases on animal biology, biochemistry, cellular physiology, anatomy and professional studies. In the second and third years, the emphasis becomes the understanding of diseases, and their causation, diagnosis, treatment and prevention. In the fourth year, a strong clinical focus is provided, which is then reinforced in fifth year through 38 weeks of core and elective clinical rotations, both in the Veterinary Medical Centre and off-campus practices.

A strong commitment to research training in veterinary sciences is provided through clinical research electives. The School of Veterinary Science has outstanding teaching and research programs encompassing all aspects of veterinary science, with particular strengths in biosecurity and infectious diseases, genetics, medicine, nutrition, Australian wildlife, farm animal and equine medicine, production and reproduction.

APPLICATION INFORMATION

For specific information on applying for a place in the program, please refer to the UQ Science Prospectus, which is updated annually (science.uq.edu.au/prospectus).

The school enrols approximately 120-130 students annually, of which, up to 40 seats are held for international students. International students must hold a student visa for the duration of their studies.

SUMMARY OF ADMISSIONS PROCEDURES

There are no specific interviews for international applicants.

International applicants for the program at UQ can submit an application directly to the university or through one of UQ's authorised International Education Representatives (future-students.uq.edu.au/find-international-representative)

Domestic students, or international students studying in Australia, may apply for entry through the Queensland Tertiary Admissions Centre (qtac.edu.au).

Successful applicants can apply to defer for one year after receiving an offer of a seat in the program.

Is a Bachelor's Degree Required? no

Is this an International School? yes

ESTIMATED TUITION

Information about fees for international students can be found on The University of Queensland Future Students website (future-students.uq.edu.au/apply/undergraduate/international/fees). Fees are subject to annual indexation (ppl.app.uq.edu.au/content/3.40.03-student-refunds).

Full-time enrolment consists of 16 units per annum or 80 units for the veterinary science program.

AVAILABLE SEATS

Domestic: 80

International: 40

VMCAS Participation: non-VMCAS

Accepts International Students? yes

APPLICATION DEADLINE

International applicants are eligible to participate in streamlined visa processing. It is recommended that international student applications are received by UQ by 30 November in the year preceding entry.

CRICOS Provider Number 00025B

ROSS UNIVERSITY SCHOOL OF VETERINARY MEDICINE

Email Address: Admissions@RossU.edu
Website: veterinary.rossu.edu

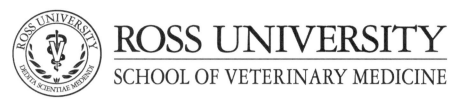

ROSS UNIVERSITY
SCHOOL OF VETERINARY MEDICINE

SCHOOL DESCRIPTION

Ross University School of Veterinary Medicine (Ross), located in St. Kitts, West Indies, offers an accredited DVM program focused on educating tomorrow's leaders and discoverers in veterinary medicine. Ross holds current accreditation from the American Veterinary Medical Association (AVMA*) and the St. Kitts and Nevis Accreditation Board. At Ross, our passion is training students to become the next generation of career-ready, compassionate veterinarians. Our 4,000+ graduates are successfully practicing veterinary medicine across the US, Canada, and beyond.

> Discover a world of possibilities in veterinary medicine at Ross.

The seven-semester pre-clinical curriculum is enhanced by hands-on clinical experience to help prepare students for the final year of clinical training at one of Ross's 32 AVMA-accredited schools in the US, UK, Canada, Australia, New Zealand, and Ireland. Ross's faculty have outstanding credentials in teaching and research and share a passion for educating the veterinarians of tomorrow. Ross operates on a three-semester per year calendar.

Each semester is 15 full academic weeks, including final exams. Ross graduates are eligible to practice veterinary medicine in all 50 states, Canada and Puerto Rico upon completion of the requisite licensing requirements. Ross students who are U.S. citizens/permanent residents and meet the Department of Education's qualifying criteria may be eligible for Federal Stafford Loans and Federal Graduate PLUS Loans.

APPLICATION INFORMATION

- Students can apply through VMCAS or directly through Ross.

EVALUATION CRITERIA

- Undergraduate cumulative grade point average (GPA)

- GPA in required pre-veterinary coursework

- Advanced science courses (Cell Biology, Genetics, Microbiology, Anatomy and Physiology, etc.)

- Graduate Record Examination (GRE) scores

- Personal essay

- Letters of recommendation from academic and/or professional references (at least one letter should be from a veterinarian)

- Extracurricular activities and accomplishments

- Personal qualities

- Personal interview

- Record of professional veterinary experience (working with animals or veterinary research) - at least 150 hours

SUMMARY OF ADMISSIONS PROCEDURES

Timetable (for VMCAS applications)

Application deadline: September 15, 2017 at 12 Midnight Eastern Time

Date interviews are held: Year-round

Date acceptances mailed: As soon as possible after the interview

School begins: Three start dates per year: September, January and May

TIMETABLE

Application deadline: None; rolling admissions

Date interviews are held: Year-round

Date acceptances mailed: As soon as possible after the interview

School begins: Three start dates per year: September, January and May

Deposit (to hold place in class): $1,000.00

Deferments: Considered

ENTRANCE REQUIREMENTS

To be considered for review by the admission committee the applicant must complete at least 48 credits of college work.

Course completion deadline: Required courses must be completed prior to enrollment.

AP credit policy: Must appear on official college transcripts.

Standardized Examinations: Results of the Graduate Record Examination (GRE) are required.

English Language Proficiency: Applicants presenting fewer than 60 upper division credits from an English language college or university must provide the official record of the scores for the Test of English as a Foreign Language (TOEFL). The minimum acceptable score is 550 on the paper-based test, or 213 on the computer-based test.

Is a Bachelor's Degree Required? no

Is this an International School? yes

ESTIMATED TUITION

Resident and Non-Resident: $18,310**

AVAILABLE SEATS

Resident and Non-Resident: 130

TEST REQUIREMENTS

Results of the Graduate Record Examination (GRE) are required.

English Language Proficiency: Applicants presenting fewer than 60 upper division credits from an English language college or university must provide the official record of the scores for the Test of English as a Foreign Language (TOEFL). The minimum acceptable score is 550 on the paper-based test, or 213 on the computer-based test.

VMCAS Participation: partial

Accepts International Students? yes

ADDITIONAL INFORMATION

Application Deadline: 9/15/2017

---

* Ross's Doctor of Veterinary Medicine degree is accredited by the AVMA COE. AVMA Council on Education. Phone: 800-248-2862 www.avma.org

**Tuition rates are subject to change

ROYAL VETERINARY COLLEGE

Email Address: admissions@rvc.ac.uk
Website: http://www.rvc.ac.uk

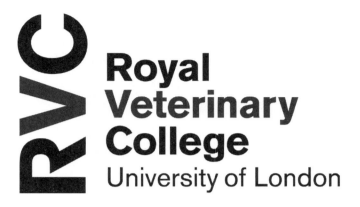

SCHOOL DESCRIPTION

The RVC has a successful record of training North American students and can count several hundred American and Canadian graduates as alumni. Founded in 1791, the RVC was the first veterinary school in the UK, and the driving force behind the establishment of the nation's veterinary profession. The first four students were admitted in January 1792, and ever since the College has been at the forefront of teaching and research in veterinary and allied sciences. The RVC was the first Veterinary School to submit a woman for membership to the Royal College of Veterinary Surgeons; become an independent veterinary school within a federal university; be accredited by the American Veterinary Medical Association; introduce a degree in Veterinary Nursing; and establish a Centre for Lifelong and Independent Veterinary Education. Today, first-class teaching and research staff, experienced in a wide range of disciplines and skills, help talented students to exploit state-of-the-art clinical facilities and laboratories to the full, maintaining the RVC's long, proud tradition of making seminal contributions to both the animal and human sciences.

> The Royal Veterinary College is at the forefront of teaching and research in veterinary and allied sciences.

We have one campus near Kings Cross/Camden Town, in central London (the Camden Campus) and one located close to the outskirts of London on a 575-acre site near Potters Bar (the Hawkshead Campus). Both offer a friendly and supportive environment and excellent facilities for teaching and learning. The Camden Campus boasts newly refurbished research laboratories, and extensive library, an anatomy museum, the London Bioscience Innovation Centre and the Beaumont-Sainsbury Animal Hospital. Accommodation, a fitness room, a restaurant and a bar, and a social learning space including a cafe are also on site and the clubs, bars, restaurants and theatres of Camden and London's West End are easily accessed on foot or by public transport. A twenty-minute walk from the Campus is the University of London whose collegiate structure incorporates the RVC. Here in the capital's university quarter, you will find some of the nation's greatest educational and research facilities.

The Hawkshead Campus is our main clinical campus with three state-of-the-art teaching hospitals on site including the largest veterinary-referral hospital in Europe. Located in rural countryside near Potters Bar, it is a 20 minute train journey from London's Kings Cross station and comprises lecture theatres, laboratories, a Learning Resources Centre (providing superb IT resources and teaching and library facilities), a Clinical Skills Centre and student housing, a refectory, sports fields, and a student-run bar. In addition to the modern journals and textbooks you will find in our libraries, the RVC has one of the best collections of old veterinary books in the world. The RVC has invested heavily in the Hawkshead Campus in recent years, developing a new Student Village with over 190 bedrooms, a new refectory for both staff and students, a state-of-the-art Teaching and Research Centre and a world-class Equine Hospital. Our working-farm is also located at this campus.

Places in RVC halls of residence are available and students from overseas are given priority. The College has a number of dedicated staff who provide academic and pastoral support to students throughout the course, and we have an active and welcoming student community.

APPLICATION INFORMATION

For specific application information (availability, deadlines, fees and VMCAS participation), please refer to our website at http://www.rvc.ac.uk/study/undergraduate/bvetmed-graduate-accelerated#panel-international-and-e-u-applicants.

Residency implications: The UK government introduced a points-based immigration system for students from non-EU countries who wish to study in the UK. For further information on entry to the UK, please refer to https://www.gov.uk/browse/visas-immigration/student-visas and to the College's web site. Students must also be able to ensure adequate financial support for the duration of their course.

SUMMARY OF ADMISSIONS PROCEDURES

Timetable

VMCAS application deadline: Friday, September 15, 2017 at 12 Midnight Eastern Time

Interview dates are arranged: October

Date interviews are held: November

Date acceptances mailed: January to March

School begins: September

Transcripts: All transcripts to VMCAS by 15 September. But aim for 1 September in case of problems.

Deposit (to hold place in class): Deposit is not required to hold the place but is required before the place can be confirmed.

Deferments: may be considered in exceptional circumstances.

EVALUATION CRITERIA

Academic performance
Animal/veterinary experience
Interview
An academic reference must be provided. Reference(s) will also be required to demonstrate experience in animal and veterinary environments.
Personal statement

ENTRANCE REQUIREMENTS

Course requirements

VMCAS applicants are normally final year or recent university graduates although students with two years pre-vet will be considered. We will also consider High School students studying AP or the International Baccalaureate. These students apply through UCAS (see our website at http://www.rvc.ac.uk/study/international-students/your-country#panel-north-america). Science graduates or applicants in the final year of a science based degree with the prerequisites may be considered for our 4 year accelerated course. Applicants who are unsuccessful in gaining a place on the four year programme may be considered for our five year programme. Required at upper level (i.e., 300-400 level): At least 8 upper-level credits in Biology/Biological Science. Examples include but are not limited to: Animal Biology, Physiology, Anatomy, Zoology, Microbiology or Genetics.

Also required (4 semester credits each): Biochemistry, Physics, Mathematics, Anatomy/Physiology, Organic Chemistry, and Biology.

Required undergraduate GPA: 3.40 or higher preferred (on 4.0 point scale).

AP credit policy: not applicable for graduate applicants.

Course completion deadline: all required courses should be completed by July of the year of admissions.

Standardized examinations: GRE General test required and must be sent to the College by 15 September. RVC institution code is 3207.

ADDITIONAL REQUIREMENTS AND CONSIDERATIONS

Applicants are also expected to have gained significant relevant work experience of handling animals. This should include work in both veterinary practice and non-clinical environments.

Supplemental Application: see website

Is a Bachelor's Degree Required? no

Is this an International School? yes

ESTIMATED TUITION

Estimated Tuition Resident: pending, see our website for further information

Estimated Tuition Contract: none

Estimated Tuition Non-Resident: pending, see our website for further information

AVAILABLE SEATS

Resident: tbc

Contract: none

Non-Resident: tbc

TEST REQUIREMENTS

Standardized examinations: GRE General test required and to be submitted to the RVC by 15 September. RVC institution code is 3207.

VMCAS Participation: partial

Accepts International Students? yes

ADDITIONAL INFORMATION

Application Deadline: 9/15/2017

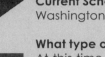

PRE-VET PROFILE: LACEY ROSE

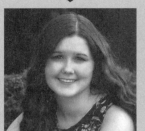

Current School Name
Washington State University

What type of veterinary medicine are you interested in pursuing, and why?
At this time I am considering a mixed practice of both small and large animals because I think it would be exciting to have such a large variety of animals to work on everyday.

What is/was your major during undergraduate school?
Animal sciences.

What are your short-term and long-term goals?
My short-term goal is to find a balance between all of the extracurricular activities I wish to participate in and the homework load that I currently have. My long-term goals are to be admitted into veterinary school and to eventually work in a large hospital with other great veterinarians.

What are you doing as an applicant/pre-vet to prepare for veterinary school?
I am currently emailing veterinary clinics back home to see if I can find an internship for the summer, and I am a part of the Honors College at Washington State University, hoping to be admitted to the seven-year veterinary medicine program they offer.

What extracurricular activities are you involved in currently?
I am involved in the Washington State University Pre-Vet Club, the Cougar Success Program (a leadership group), and I hope to be working in a research lab later in the semester.

How old were you when you first became interested in being a veterinarian?
I have dreamed of becoming a veterinarian since I was five years old.

Please describe your various experiences in preparation for applying to veterinary school.
I have volunteered at the local animal shelter for the past two years, and I have owned two cats for about ten years.

What characteristics are you looking for in a veterinary school?
Preferably one that is in or close to the state of Washington and one that allows students to receive a lot of hands-on experience in and out of the classroom.

What advice do you have for other pre-veterinary students?
Get involved as soon as possible with a veterinary clinic.

UNIVERSITY OF SASKATCHEWAN
WESTERN COLLEGE OF VETERINARY MEDICINE

Email Address: wcvm.admissions@usask.ca
Website: http://www.usask.ca/wcvm

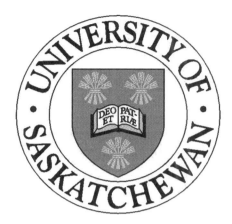

SCHOOL DESCRIPTION

The Western College of Veterinary Medicine is located in the city of Saskatoon, which has a population of about 265,000 and is the major urban center in central Saskatchewan. The city is also the major commercial center for central and northern Saskatchewan and is served by 2 national airlines with direct connections to all major centers in Canada.

The Western College of Veterinary Medicine is one of the few veterinary colleges where all health sciences and agriculture are offered on the same campus. The college is devoted to undergraduate education and has a reputation in Canada and in the northwestern United States for educating veterinarians who are well-rounded in general veterinary medicine and have good practical backgrounds. It has one of the best field-service caseloads in North America.

> The Western College of Veterinary Medicine has one of the best field-service caseloads in North America.

APPLICATION INFORMATION

For specific application information (availability, deadlines, fees, and VMCAS participation), please refer to the contact information listed above.

Residency implications: Currently, 78 students are selected for quota positions from Alberta, British Columbia, Manitoba, Saskatchewan, and the Yukon, Nunavut, and Northwest Territories. Special consideration is given to self identified individuals of aboriginal origin. Residents of foreign countries are not considered.

SUMMARY OF ADMISSIONS PROCEDURES

Timetable

Application deadline: December 1

Reference deadline: February 15

Date interviews are held: May–June

Date acceptances mailed: on or before July 1

School begins: late August

Deposit (to hold place in class): none required.

Deferments: not considered.

EVALUATION CRITERIA

The 3-part admission procedure consists of an assessment of academic ability, a personal interview, and an overall assessment of the application file.

% weight

Grades 60%

Interview* 40%

* Interview selection is based entirely on academic performance.

ENTRANCE REQUIREMENTS

Required undergraduate GPA: a minimum cumulative average of 75% is required.

Course completion deadline: prerequisite courses must be completed by the time of entry into the program.

Standardized examinations: none required.

PREREQUISITES FOR ADMISSION

Course Description	Number of Hours/Credits	Necessity
English	6	Required
Physics	3	Required
Biology	6	Required
Genetics	3	Required
Introductory Chemistry	6	Required
Organic Chemistry	3	Required
Mathematics or Statistics	6	Required
Biochemistry	3	Required
Microbiology	3	Required
Electives	21	Required

Reference Forms: Two required—one from a veterinarian and one from an individual with an agricultural- or animal-related background.

Additional Requirements/Information: Space is provided on the application form to nominate referees to support the application. Referees will be contacted directly and asked to complete the reference form online.

ADDITIONAL REQUIREMENTS AND CONSIDERATIONS

Animal/veterinary work experience, motivation, and knowledge

Maturity

Leadership

Communication skills

Is a Bachelor's Degree Required? no

Is this an International School? no

ESTIMATED TUITION

Estimated Tuition Resident: $9,933.97

Estimated Tuition Contract: $9,933.97

Estimated Tuition Non-Resident: $9,933.97

AVAILABLE SEATS

Resident: 20

Contract: 57

Non-Resident: 1

TEST REQUIREMENTS

None

VMCAS Participation: non-VMCAS

Accepts International Students? no

ADDITIONAL INFORMATION

Application Deadline: 12/1/2017 for fall 2018 entry

ST. GEORGE'S UNIVERSITY

Email Address: SGUEnrolment@sgu.edu
Website: http://www.sgu.edu

St. George's University

SCHOOL DESCRIPTION

Having received full accreditation by the AVMA COE in 2011, St. George's University School of Veterinary Medicine is proud of its academic excellence exemplified by its breadth of highly regarded education, unprecedented student support services, and internationally recognized faculty. The core mission of the University is creating excellent academic programs within an international setting where students and faculty are actively recruited from around the world. St. Georges University has drawn faculty and students from over 140 countries, assembling a diverse community of disparate cultural and educational backgrounds.

> SGU prepares its students for leadership, life-long success and service in a constantly changing world.

Located on the southwest corner of the Caribbean island of Grenada, St. George's shoreline location offers its growing student body a serene environment in which to live, learn and create a worldwide network of friends and colleagues. Along with St. George's state-of-the-art facilities, complete with a large animal facility and, marine station, and the SGU Small Animal Clinic, St. George's University School of Veterinary Medicine prepares its students for leadership, life-long success and service in a constantly changing world.

Over 6,000 students from throughout the world are enrolled in the University's School of Medicine, School of Veterinary Medicine, School of Arts and Sciences or graduate programs which include a CEPH-accredited MPH and MBA program. SGU students also benefit from world-renowned international academic partnerships with universities, hospitals and other educational and scientific institutions.

The veterinary medical program is delivered with a number of entry options: the seven-, six- and five-year programs which begin with the preveterinary medical sciences and an option to enter directly into the four-year veterinary medical program. This enables students flexible entry points depending upon their academic backgrounds. Students accepted into the preveterinary medical sciences are placed in the appropriate program option (either the seven-, six- or five-year program track) according to their academic background and are enrolled in the veterinary medical program for five to seven years. Applicants accepted directly into the veterinary medical sciences generally complete the program in four years.

The DVM program is conducted on the University's main campus on the True Blue peninsula of Grenada, West Indies, except for the final year which is the clinical year spent at an affiliated AVMA-accredited School of Veterinary Medicine. These schools are located in the United States, Canada, United Kingdom, Ireland, and Australia.

APPLICATION INFORMATION

As a member of the Association of American Veterinary Medical Colleges (AAVMC) the School of Veterinary Medicine participates in the AAVMC's centralized Veterinary Medical College Application Service (VMCAS). Aspiring veterinary medical students have the option of applying to the January 2018 or August 2018 entering class through the VMCAS 2017 application cycle. To learn more or apply go to http://aavmc.org/Students -Applicants-and-Advisors.aspx.

PREREQUISITES FOR ADMISSION

Course Description	Number of Hours/Credits	Necessity
General Biology or Zoology with Lab	8	Required
Inorganic Chemistry (general or Physical) with lab	8	Required
Organic Chemistry with lab	4	Required
Biochemistry	3	Required
Genetics	3	Required
Physics with lab	4	Required
Calculus, Computer Science or Statistics	3	Required
English	3	Required

If you are not applying through VMCAS we encourage you to apply online through the SGU website at www.sgu.edu/apply-now/index.html and track your application through Self Service Admission. As an alternative, you can still download a paper copy to print and complete manually.

SUMMARY OF ADMISSIONS PROCEDURES

Application Deadlines for August and January Matriculation: The Committee on Admission utilizes a rolling admission policy in the School of Veterinary Medicine; therefore, applications are accepted and reviewed on an ongoing basis. The final deadline for receipt of direct (non-VMCAS) applications and all supporting documentation is April 15 of the current year for the August class, and November 15 of the preceding year for the January class. Prospective candidates should note that the entering classes are highly competitive and those applications completed early have the advantage of being reviewed at the beginning of the admission process. The time necessary to secure official transcripts, standardized test scores, and letters of recommendation should be taken into consideration. The Committee reserves the right to defer an application to the following semester if there are no available seats.

The Office of Admission will acknowledge receipt of a candidate's application within two weeks of its arrival. A candidate will be informed of any required supporting documents missing at that time. Within one month after receipt of all application materials, a candidate will receive notice that the application is complete and being reviewed to determine whether an interview will be granted.

The Office of Admission encourages candidates who have been approved for an interview to request interviews in Grenada, and will schedule one upon the applicant's request. The University recognizes that financial considerations may prevent many candidates who reside at great distances from Grenada from choosing this option.

Interviews, therefore, may be conducted in the United States, the United Kingdom, Canada, the Caribbean, or other locations that best serve the diverse applicant pool. Candidates are advised that being granted an interview is no guarantee of acceptance; the interview itself plays a significant part in the decision by the Committee on Admission. Applicants are notified of the decision of the Committee on Admission. A record of the notification is kept for one year.

ENTRANCE REQUIREMENTS

The requirements for direct entry into the four-year DVM program vary depending on the educational system of your home country. What is required for all applicants is completion of secondary school, a period of farm experience or time spent in a veterinary practice, and possession of a bachelors degree from an accredited University or 60 credit hours.

Specific undergraduate coursework (or its equivalent) is required as part of the preveterinary medical sciences requirements for admission.

Two letters of recommendation. In order of importance to the Committee on Admission, these are the categories:

a. A veterinarian with whom you have worked

b. A university professor (or, for those applying for the preveterinary program, a teacher)

c. A preveterinary advisor committee, or an advisor/counselor.

One essay: A personal statement discussing the significant factors which led to your decision to pursue a career in veterinary medicine, and how you see yourself using this career to make a difference in the world (maximum 1500 words).

Applicants from North America

A completed bachelors degree from an accredited university is required for direct entry into the four-year veterinary medical program. A candidate may apply before completion of the degree. Under exceptional circumstances a candidate may be considered with 60 undergraduate credit hours.

Standardized Examination: Candidates must submit scores by the corresponding application deadlines (see below) on the Graduate Record Examination or alternatively on the MCAT. (Our GRE Code is 7153; MCAT code 21303.)

Applicants from Other Systems of Education

For direct entry into the four-year DVM program, a bachelors degree with a strong science background is required.

Applicants with passes at the Advanced Level of the General Certificate of Education will be assessed individually and will be considered for appropriate entry into the five-year DVM program. Generally, A Level students with the appropriate courses and grades matriculate into the five-year veterinary medical program.

If English is not the principal language, the applicant must have achieved a score in the Test of English as a Foreign Language (TOEFL) of at least 600 points, 250 points computer-based or 100 points internet-based.

Is a Bachelor's Degree Required? yes

Is this an International School? yes

ESTIMATED TUITION

Estimated Tuition Resident: average $42,500 per year

Estimated Tuition Contract: 0

Estimated Tuition Non-Resident: average $42,500 per year

AVAILABLE SEATS

Each class consists of 110 students. No preference is given to applicant's place of residence.

TEST REQUIREMENTS

Standardized Examination: Candidates must submit scores by the corresponding application deadlines (see below) on the Graduate Record Examination or alternatively on the MCAT. (Our GRE Code is 7153; MCAT code 21303.)

VMCAS Participation: partial

Accepts International Students? yes

ADDITIONAL INFORMATION

Dual Degree Programs

Combined DVM/MPH, MSc, and MBA degree programs are available. Applications can be submitted online directly through the SGU website at www.sgu.edu or via the VMCAS application system. If you have questions about the application process, please call one of our admission advisors at 1 (800) 899-6337, ext 1280.

Application Deadline: 9/15/2017

UNIVERSITY OF SYDNEY

Email: vet.science@sydney.edu.au
Website: http://sydney.edu.au/vetscience

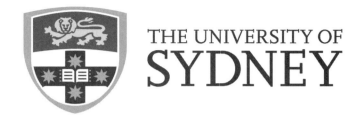

SCHOOL INFORMATION

As Australia's first university, the University of Sydney's reputation spans more than 160 years. We are regularly ranked in the top 0.3% of universities worldwide. We teach more than 50,000 bright minds, with 10,000 international students from more than 145 countries. We've taught 145 Olympians, 6 prime ministers, 2 Nobel laureates, 3 astronauts,110 Rhodes scholars and 1 Pulitzer Prize winner. When you come to study at the University of Sydney, you become part of an inspiring network of leading academics, and distinguished graduates and alumni.

> The University of Sydney's School of Veterinary Science delivers inspirational and innovative student-centered teaching

Located only ten minutes by bus from the heart of the Sydney business district, the main Camperdown campus provides easy access to Sydney's vibrant social scene, Sydney harbour and surrounds.

One of the best aspects of studying at the University of Sydney is that it is located in the most beautiful city in the 'down-under' country of Australia, which is a young, modern and dynamic city.

The Sydney School of Veterinary Science was established in 1910 and is the oldest continuing School of its kind in Australia. We are an international leader in veterinary and animal education and ranked as Australia's top university and equal 9th in the world for veterinary science in the latest QS World University Rankings (2016). We received a score of 5/5 from Excellence in Research for Australia (ERA) for veterinary science research. The School delivers inspirational and innovative student-centered teaching emphasizing life-long, evidence-based learning whilst also providing clinical and research excellence through creative, collaborative programs.

We maintain teaching hospitals on both the inner-city Camperdown campus and the rural Camden campus, where you will work with veterinarians in a clinical teaching and learning environment. Referral and primary accession cases are seen at both sites. The University Veterinary Teaching Hospital at Camden also provides veterinary services to farms in the region, while the Wildlife Health and Conservation Clinic provides veterinary services to sick and injured Australian native wildlife; reptiles; and avian, aquatic and exotic pets. A wide range of companion animals, farm animals, racing animals, exotic and native species are seen. We have a strong global network of more than 5,000 alumni across the veterinary, agricultural and public health sectors, including graduates in North America and Canada. Our active student societies, including VetSoc and the Camden Farms Society, ensure a rich and rewarding experience both in and out of the classroom.

The Doctor of Veterinary Medicine (DVM) program aims to produce career ready graduates with excellent fundamental knowledge and skills in managing animal health and disease; and in protecting and advancing animal, human and environmental health and welfare locally and globally. Clinical exposure, clinical skills training and animal handling commence in the first semester and continue throughout the course. The program culminates in a lecture-free capstone experience year where you will be placed as an intern in a variety of different veterinary clinics and in a wide range of locations, including rotations in the University Teaching Hospitals at Sydney and Camden and in our Wildlife Health and Conservation Clinic.

The DVM program will equip you with the knowledge and skills to choose from many career options as a veterinary professional participating in the care and welfare of animals. Completion of the course will provide you with a wide knowledge of the principles associated with every aspect of health and disease in animals—domestic and wild.

ENTRY PATHWAYS

The University of Sydney has two pathways for you to study veterinary medicine:

1. *Undergraduate applicants:* You can apply for entry into a combined six-year Bachelor of Veterinary Biology/Doctor of Veterinary Medicine (BVetBiol/DVM) on the basis of your secondary school results (plus additional selection criteria). The BVetBiol/DVM commences with two years of undergraduate study in the Bachelor of Veterinary Biology and if you perform well you will be eligible to progress to the Doctor of Veterinary Medicine in years 3-6. Undergraduate applications must be direct to the University.

2. *Graduate applicants:* If you have completed a bachelor degree, and have completed the prerequisite subjects* you can apply for entry into the four-year DVM program. Graduate DVM applications are through VMCAS.

*Prerequisites for the DVM are the successful completion of at least one semester of study in general chemistry (physical and inorganic), organic chemistry, biology and biochemistry. University of Sydney units of study that meet the prerequisite requirements are provided as examples of the content that all applicants are assumed to have, these can be found on: http://sydney.edu.au/courses/doctor-of-veterinary-medicine

ADMISSION REQUIREMENTS

Academic Performance:
1. If you are applying as an undergraduate for the BVetBiol/DVM, you will be assessed on the basis of your academic achievement in your final year of secondary education (Year 12 or equivalent) or your tertiary stud-

ies from a recognized University. Minimum GPA required for BVetBiol/DVM entry is 2.80 on a 4.00 scale, and you must demonstrate an aptitude for science-based study.

2. If you are applying as a graduate for the DVM, you will be assessed on the basis of your completed bachelor degree from the University of Sydney or another accredited institution, along with your relevant work experience. Minimum GPA required for DVM entry is 2.80 on a 4.00 scale. You must have successfully completed the prerequisite subjects, which can be found on http://sydney.edu.au/vetscience/dvm/prerequisites.shtml.

3. *Additional requirements and considerations:* You are expected to have gained relevant work experience and animal handling. You must demonstrate your relevant work experience in your application. For graduate entry, the minimum work experience is four weeks, undertaken within two years of the application date.

PRACTICAL EXPERIENCE

During the inter-semester and intra-semester breaks you will be required to undertake, placements for preparatory clinical and animal husbandry experience. The final year is free of lectures, and instead, you will participate in practice-based activities and the management and care of patients.

PROFESSIONAL RECOGNITION

Sydney graduates are immediately eligible for registration for practice with the Veterinary Practitioners Board in each Australian state and territory and are recognised by the Royal College of Veterinary Surgeons in the United Kingdom and the American Veterinary Medical Association.

APPLICATION INFORMATION

Applications for the Undergraduate Bachelor of Veterinary Biology/Doctor of Veterinary Medicine must be made directly to the University via http://sydney.edu.au/courses. For the graduate entry DVM, you can apply through VMCAS or directly to the University. Please note, if applying directly, you will need to complete the Supplementary application form available via the University's Courses website: http://sydney.edu.au/courses/doctor-of-veterinary-medicine.

You may also be interested in obtaining information about the University of Sydney from one of these University representatives: http://sydney.edu.au/future-students /international/undergraduate/find-an-agent.php

VMCAS and Direct Application Deadline: Applicants need to check the website for the 2017 opening and closing dates:

http://sydney.edu.au/courses/bachelor-of-veterinary -biology-and-doctor-of-veterinary-medicine

http://sydney.edu.au/courses/programs/postgrad-veterinary -medicine/doctor-of-veterinary-medicine

It should be noted the semester for the four-year DVM program commences in early February each year.

NEW ENTRANTS

Bachelor of Veterinary Biology/DVM:

Australian Resident: 40

International: 35

Doctor of Veterinary Medicine (Graduate entry):

Australian Resident: 22

International: 27

TUITION FEES 2018(INDICATIVE FEES)

Information on tuition fees can be found on the website relating to each degree:

http://sydney.edu.au/courses/bachelor-of-veterinary -biology-and-doctor-of-veterinary-medicine

http://sydney.edu.au/courses/doctor-of-veterinary -medicine

UTRECHT UNIVERSITY

Email: secretariaat.bic.vet@uu.nl
Website: www.uu.nl/vet

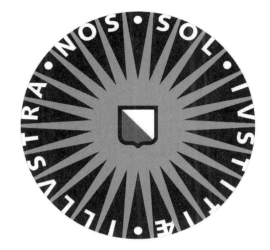

SHORT HISTORY

In 1821 a state veterinary school was founded in Utrecht. Almost a century later, in 1918, the school acquired the status of an institution of higher learning and in 1925 it was incorporated into the State University of Utrecht and thereby became the first and until to date the only Faculty of Veterinary Medicine in the Netherlands. Utrecht University, founded in 1636, is one of the 14 universities in the Netherlands. The faculty of Veterinary Medicine is now one of the 6 faculties of Utrecht University and is located at campus site De Uithof just outside the city of Utrecht. The Faculty of Veterinary Medicine is housed in modern and spacious buildings on a total surface of 60.000 m.

> Utrecht University is one of the 14 universities in the Netherlands and is located at campus site De Uithof.

ORGANISATION AND STAFF

The faculty encompasses 8 departments with specialized facilities, a Faculty Office and a number of general services (e.g. leaning environment with audio-visual units and the library, pharmacy, experimental farms, museum, student computer rooms etc). The faculty has an academic staff of 418 fte, including 32 full professors and an administrative and support staff of 484 fte. Most staff members can communicate well in English and most lecturers have experience in teaching veterinary medicine in the English language.

VETERINARY EDUCATION

Admission of students to the 6-year veterinary training programme (taught in Dutch) is limited to 225 each year, resulting in a total of 1400 students. The veterinary curriculum leads to the 'dierenarts' degree (Doctor of Veterinary Medicine, DVM). In September 2007 the veterinary education under a Bachelor - Master (3+3 years) structure started. The 1st year of the master programme started in September 2010.

RESEARCH AND POSTGRADUATE EDUCATION

Research at the faculty of Veterinary Medicine is the responsibility of the Institute for Veterinary Research (IVR). Research which is conducted as part of PhD programmes is linked to one of the research programmes of the IVR.

QUALITY OF EDUCATION

The faculty of Veterinary Medicine is accredited by the American Veterinary Medical Association (AVMA) and Canadian Veterinary Medical Association (CVMA) since 1973, the European Association of Establishments of Veterinary Education and the Dutch and Flemish Accreditation Organization.

INFORMATION ABOUT THE ADMISSION TO THE FACULTY OF VETERINARY MEDICINE FOR INTERNATIONAL STUDENTS

Special rules apply for the study of Veterinary Medicine. The Dutch Ministry of Education has declared the so-called 'numerus fixes' applicable to the study of Veterinary Medicine. This entails that only a limited amount of students is admitted each year. The number of admission requests largely exceeds the number of allocations. Those restrictions affect both Dutch and international students. The available places are assigned by selection through interviews or drawing lots.

APPLICATION AND DRAWING LOTS

Each year the minister of Education and Science determines the number of students that can be admitted to the study of Veterinary Medicine. At this moment the number is 225. In order to take part in the lottery for placement, you need to complete an application form via Internet (start with website: http://www.uu.nl/bachelors/en/limited-enrolment-programmes-dutch) and send this in before May 15th. The deadline for the selection interviews was 15 January 2016.

If you do not apply you cannot participate in drawing lots.

NON-DUTCH DIPLOMAS

Non-Dutch diplomas have to be evaluated and compared with the Dutch equivalent diplomas. This evaluation takes time and can result in the fact that you have to take supplementary exams before being accepted for the lottery. Information about the evaluation of your diplomas can be obtained at:
Utrecht University, Admissions Office
P.O. Box 80 125, 3508 TC Utrecht, the Netherlands
Phone: +31 30 253 7000
Visiting Address: Heidelberglaan 6, Utrecht – De Uithof

DUTCH LANGUAGE EXAM

If the result of the lottery is favorable, then - prior to admission to the study of Veterinary Medicine - you have to prove your (sufficient) knowledge of the Dutch language. This is a requirement under the Dutch law because the education is in the Dutch language. The owner of a non-Dutch diploma therefore has to pass the exam "Dutch as Second Language program 2" ('Staatsexamen Nederlands als Tweede Taal, programma 2'), or the Certificate of Dutch as a foreign language 'Certificaat Nederlands als Vreemde Taal: 'Profiel Academische Taalvaardigheid' (PAT) or "Profiel Taalvaardigheid Hoger Onderwijs" (PTHO)' before being admitted. More information about language requirements, courses and examinations can be found through http://www.uu.nl/bachelors/en/limited-enrolment-programmes-dutch under Entry requirements.

TUITION FEES AND SCHOLARSHIPS

The tuition fee depends on your nationality and the programme you register for:

Nationality Programme Tuition 2015-2016

EU/EEA: Bachelor's and Master's programmes: €1,951

Non EU/EEA BSc Veterinary Medicine: €20,000

MSc Veterinary Medicine: €20,700

Information about grants, loans etc. can be found at http://www.uu.nl/bachelors/en/grants-and-scholarships-0.

RESIDENCE PERMIT

Every international student who wants to receive academic education in the Netherlands needs a residence permit. More information can be obtained at the International Office.

DOCUMENTATION

When requesting admission, the following documents have to be sent to the Admissions Office (see above):

- Your passport copy
- A certified copy of your diploma, OR a certified statement of your school, with the name of the diploma you will obtain and when, and the subjects in which you will be examined
- A certified copy of your transcript
- Official translations of your diploma and transcript (if documents are not in Dutch, English, French, German or Spanish)
- Proof of your proficiency in Dutch

For further information about the admission to the study of Veterinary Medicine please contact:
Study adviser
Faculty of Veterinary Medicine
Department of Educational and Student Affairs
PO Box 80163, 3508 TD Utrecht, the Netherlands
E-mail: osz@vet.uu.nl

FIRST-YEAR PROFILE: JESSICA BECHER

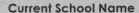

Current School Name
CVM at North Carolina State University

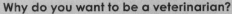

Why do you want to be a veterinarian?
I want to help relieve suffering in this world and play a role in the scientific community to make a large-scale impact on the lives of both humans and animals.

What are your short-term and long-term goals?
My short-term goal is to make it through veterinary school with the best experiences and academic standing I can get. For long-term, I'm thinking of becoming involved with laboratory animal medicine.

What did you do as an applicant to prepare for applying to veterinary school?
I shadowed in multiple fields of veterinary medicine and made good contacts. I intentionally took a gap year to get more hands-on experience in a small animal clinic and earn some money before applying to veterinary school, which worked out great for me. I have far better venipuncture skills than I ever got just shadowing and interning. I also challenged myself with hard science-based classes in undergrad.

What advice would you give to applicants or those considering applying to veterinary school?
Take physiology and cell biology before going to veterinary school. You will be at a disadvantage first year if you do not, even though they were not required for my vet school at my time of application. Also, get research experience even if you do not plan on pursuing anything like that in the future. It never hurts and always looks great on applications. Plus, you might enjoy it.

What helped make the transition to veterinary school easier for you?
Having taken hard science classes in my undergrad and learning to time manage before coming to veterinary school were honestly what made my transition to vet school easier.

What is your advice on student debt?
It is inevitable, daunting, crushing, and sometimes better to just not stress over in addition to everything else you have to stress over. But you didn't want to be a veterinarian for the money, now did you? (Because if you are pursuing it for money, you are sorely in the wrong career path.)

What are you most excited about learning in veterinary school?
Anatomy is my favorite. It is challenging because it goes at such a fast pace on multiple species, but I find it fascinating to compare species differences.

VETAGRO SUP

Email Address: international@vetagro-sup.fr
Website: http://www.vetagro-sup.fr

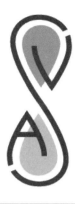

VetAgro Sup

SCHOOL DESCRIPTION

VetAgro Sup was born on January 1, 2010 from the merger of the National Veterinary School of Lyon (the oldest veterinary institution established in the world in 1761), the National School of agricultural engineers in Clermont-Ferrand and the National School of Veterinary Services.

Institute of Higher Education and Research in food, animal health, agricultural sciences and the environment, VetAgro Sup operates on both Auvergne and Rhône-Alpes regions and ranks first of its objectives training of veterinarians and engineers, production of knowledge and support for economic, social and public actors in the areas of food, animal health and welfare, agricultural sciences and the environment. VetAgro Sup trains students around multiple veterinary and agricultural occupations (animal health, public health, protection and animal safety, environmental protection, nutrition and food science, etc.).

> VetAgro Sup trains students around multiple veterinary and agricultural occupations.

This great institution was the first French structure created to train both agricultural engineers and veterinary doctors. This model is consistent with international models (university with two colleges), reinforcing the Structure international readability.

With 1,200 students (700 undergraduate vet students) and 120 faculty members gathered in this adventure, VetAgro Sup proposes a set of high-level training in the field of life, legible and competitive national, European and international. The veterinary teaching program is approved by AVMA and EAEVE.

The veterinary campus Lyon (Marcy l'Etoile) and the Agricultural Campus Clermont (Lempdes) are both valued because they offer recognized frameworks for the development of teaching and research. Benefits and services are available to companies and institutional and professional partners: laboratory analysis, medical devices, advice and expertise. Partner authorities (regions Rhône-Alpes and Auvergne, Lyon and Clermont Community, and departments of the Rhone and Puy-de-Dôme) here find a new link for the development of their competitiveness, their scientific potential and their international attractiveness.

FOR INFORMATION ON APPLYING TO VETAGRO SUP:

VetAgro Sup
College of Veterinary Medicine
1 Avenue Bourgelat
69280 Marcy L'Etoile, FRANCE
Phone: 04 78 87 25 25
Email: international@vetagro-sup.fr
Website: http://www.vetagro-sup.fr

AAVMC AFFILIATE MEMBER
VETERINARY MEDICAL SCHOOLS
Non–AVMA/COE Accredited

UNIVERSITY OF ADELAIDE

Email: avs_enquiries@adelaide.edu.au
Website: www.adelaide.edu.au

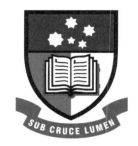

SCHOOL DESCRIPTION

The School of Animal and Veterinary Sciences at the University of Adelaide is located in South Australia. The University of Adelaide is a world-class tertiary education and research institution committed to delivering high-quality and distinct learning, teaching and research experiences. The University was established in 1874 and is consistently ranked in the top 1% of universities worldwide. It is a member of the Group of Eight, a coalition of Australia's foremost research intensive universities. The University constitutes a vibrant and diverse community with over 25,000 students and over 3,500 members of staff across our three main campuses (North Terrace, Roseworthy and Waite).

> The University of Adelaide is is consistently ranked in the top 1% of universities worldwide.

The School of Animal and Veterinary Sciences is based at the Roseworthy Campus, which is located approximately 30 miles (50 kilometres) north of Adelaide. Australia's first agricultural college was established at Roseworthy, in 1883. Since its establishment, the Australian agricultural industry has recognised Roseworthy Agricultural College as the premier teaching facility for the sector and close partnerships with industry and government research groups have always been a feature of Roseworthy's development. In 1991, the Roseworthy Agricultural College joined forces with the University of Adelaide. The Bachelor of Science (BSc) (Animal Science) has been taught at the campus since 2004 and the veterinary program commenced in 2008.

Roseworthy Campus is located on a 1600 ha property and includes a working farm on which students gain practical experience and training. In addition, our leading-edge Veterinary Health Centre (which includes the Companion Animal Health Centre, Equine Health and Performance Centre, Production Animal Health Centre and Veterinary Diagnostic Laboratories), provides exceptional services to the public and offers students in the Doctor of Veterinary Medicine (DVM) program real-world experience.

The campus is currently home to over 100 staff and approximately 650 students, including undergraduates, and post-graduates in both coursework and higher degree by research (Masters and PhD). The campus is a vibrant and exciting centre for undergraduate teaching, post-graduate training and clinical service and is fast becoming the major animal and veterinary research centre for the State.

PROGRAM OVERVIEW

At the University of Adelaide, the veterinary science program is comprised of two degrees: the BSc (Veterinary Bioscience) and the DVM. Students satisfactorily completing the undergraduate degree will gain direct entry into the postgraduate program and completion of both degrees (6 years in total) is required to register as a veterinarian.

The veterinary science program at the University of Adelaide has been granted accreditation by the Australasian Veterinary Boards Council (AVBC), the Veterinary Surgeons' Board of Hong Kong, and the Royal College of Veterinary Surgeons (UK). Graduates from this program are eligible for registration as veterinarians in all states and territories of Australia, New Zealand, Hong Kong, Singapore, South Africa and the United

Kingdom. The program also has affiliation membership with the Association of American Veterinary Medical Colleges.

APPLICATION INFORMATION

For specific application information please refer to the contact details listed above.

Residency implications: 60 domestic (Commonwealth supported places) and 20 international places.

Required academic grades:

Bachelor of Science (Veterinary Bioscience) – International Applicants

Academic entry requirements for standard qualifications are as follows:
- Australian Tertiary Admissions Rank (ATAR) – minimum 90
- International Baccalaureate (IB) – minimum 31
- Grade Point Average (GPA) – minimum of 5.0 (on a 7.0 scale)
- SAT (US) – minimum 1410

Other qualifications, including international qualifications, will be considered on their individual merits; further information is available through the degree finder on the University of Adelaide website (http://www.adelaide.edu.au/degree-finder/bscpv_bscaspv.html).

Course completion deadline: Prerequisite courses must be completed by 31st December.

Doctor of Veterinary Medicine – International Applicants
- Minimum GPA: At the discretion of the Admissions Committee

Credit policy: Students may be credited with advanced standing (status/exemption) for courses already completed at another institution and therefore may be eligible for entry into 2nd year of the BSc (Veterinary Bioscience) or 1st year of the DVM. Courses must appear on official college transcripts and be equivalent to the corresponding courses at the University of Adelaide.

Course completion deadline: Prerequisite courses must be completed by 31st December.

ADDITIONAL REQUIREMENTS AND CONSIDERATIONS

Supplemental application required:

Bachelor of Science (Veterinary Bioscience) – International Applicants

Prescribed questionnaire: To gain entry into the BSc (Veterinary Bioscience) program, applicants should be able to demonstrate an informed interest in veterinary science, animals and their welfare, and articulate a clear understanding of, and commitment to, the breadth and intensity of training which is required in a veterinary program.

Applicants must submit the Prescribed questionnaire and supporting statements (including references) by the closing date. The questionnaire includes the following components:
- Details of animal husbandry and veterinary experiences
- Personal statement demonstrating their interest in a career in the veterinary profession, references
- Extracurricular and community service activities.

Doctor of Veterinary Medicine – International Applicants

Applicants must submit to the University the Self-Assessment Checklist on skills learned in extramural studies accompanied by a 1-2 page description of how these skills were acquired.

Inherent Requirements:

There are inherent requirements associated with the BSc (Veterinary Bioscience) and DVM programs that prospective students need to be aware of before applying. Further details can be found at http://www.adelaide.edu.au/degree-finder/dvetm_drvetmedi.html

SUMMARY OF ADMISSIONS PROCEDURES

Prerequisite information

Bachelor of Science (Veterinary Bioscience) – International Applicants

Mathematics and Chemistry

English Language Requirements (if applicable)

Doctor of Veterinary Medicine – International Applicants

BSc (Veterinary Bioscience) from the University of Adelaide or equivalent.

English Language Requirements (if applicable)

ADMISSION INFORMATION

Bachelor of Science (Veterinary Bioscience) – International Applicants

Application deadlines: Applications can be received on an ongoing basis throughout the year. The final deadline is 30th September.

Interview dates: Questionnaires will be assessed as soon as possible after submission and eligible applicants will be invited to participate in an online interview. Dates and times for the interview will be negotiated between the School and the applicant.

Date acceptances mailed: Allow 2 weeks once final academic results have been received and interviews have been conducted.

School begins: March

Deferments: Up to one year

Transfer students: Yes

Evaluation Criteria: Selection for the interview process will be based on the assessment of the questionnaire. Applicants who are successful in gaining an interview will be ranked for an offer, based on a combination of scores from the following two components:

Academic Results: 50%
Interview Results: 50%

Doctor of Veterinary Medicine – International Applicants

Application Deadlines: Application can be receive on an ongoing basis throughout the year. The final deadline is 30th September.

Date acceptances mailed: Allow 2 weeks once final academic results have been received and Self-Assessment Checklist has been reviewed.

School begins: March

Deferments: Up to one year

Transfer students: Yes

Evaluation Criteria: Applicants academic transcript, grades and Self-Assessment Checklist will be assessed to determine if they are eligible and will be ranked based on their academic grades.

2016 ADMISSIONS SUMMARY

Number of applicants:

	BSc (Veterinary Bioscience)	DVM
Domestic	424	52
International	13	6
Total	437	58

Number of new entrants:

	BSc (Veterinary Bioscience)	DVM
Domestic	60	52
International	4	6
Total	64	58

EXPENSES FOR THE 2016 ACADEMIC YEAR

Tuition & Fees:

Bachelor of Science (Veterinary Bioscience)

Domestic Students (Commonwealth supported place): $9,975 per year

International Students: $58,000 per year

Doctor of Veterinary Medicine

Domestic Students (Commonwealth supported place): $10,600 per year

International Students: $58,000 per year

Scholarships: Information regarding International student scholarships can be found at http://international.adelaide.edu.au/choosing/scholarships

ENTRANCE REQUIREMENTS

Admitted students fall into two categories: Domestic (Commonwealth supported place) and International. Applicants must verify their residency status on application.

CENTRAL LUZON STATE UNIVERSITY*

Email Address: clsu@clsu.edu.ph
Website: http://clsucvsm.edu.ph

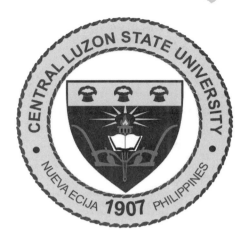

SCHOOL DESCRIPTION

Central Luzon State University (CLSU) is located on a 658-hectare sprawling main campus in the Science City of Muñoz, which is located 150 kilometers north of Manila. It also has a more than 1000-hectare site for ranch type buffalo production and forestry development up the hills of Carranglan town, in northern Nueva Ecija, 40 kilometers away from the main campus. The University is the lead agency of the Muñoz Science Community and the seat of the Regional Research and Development Center in Central Luzon. To date, CLSU is one of the premier institutions of agriculture in Southeast Asia known for its breakthrough researches in aquaculture (pioneer in the sex reversal of Tilapia), ruminants, crops, orchard, and water management researches.

> For many years, DVM graduates from CVSM have consistently topped the Veterinary Licensure Examinations in the country.

The College of Veterinary Science and Medicine (CVSM) was established in 1978 through Republic Act No. 4067 enacted into law by Congress in 1964. Subsequently, CVSM offered the first ladderized veterinary curriculum in the Philippines: Bachelor of Science in Animal Husbandry (first 4 years) and Doctor of Veterinary Medicine (6 years). This was designed to produce veterinarians adept not only in disease control and prevention but in animal production as well. For many years, DVM graduates from CVSM have consistently topped the Veterinary Licensure Examinations in the country. This excellent performance has made the Philippine Commission on Higher Education (CHED) and the Professional Regulation Commission (PRC) to recognize the CVSM as one of the Top Performing Veterinary Colleges in the country. In 2009, CHED awarded the college the title, Center of Excellence in Veterinary Medicine.

APPLICATION INFORMATION

The following are the admission requirements for both undergraduate and graduate programs:

UNDERGRADUATE PROGRAM

1. Must have a GPA of 2.25 or better. Second courser must have at least 2.50 or better.
2. Must have taken a minimum of 40 units of general education courses.
3. Must not have a grade of "5".
4. Grades of "4" or "INC" must be removed or completed upon filing of application.
5. Must qualify in the online exam and panel interview conducted by the college admission committee.
6. Submission of duly accomplished application form with:
   A. four (4) 2x2 pictures (studio taken only)
   B. certification of grades (1st and 2nd semester)

For Transferees
1. Applicants must meet all the prescribed admission requirements of the University/College and the course applied for:
   a. Must qualify in the University/College Admission Test
   b. Must have complete and valid credentials
      (a) Copy of birth certificate
      (b) Two 2"x2" colored ID pictures

(c) Certificate of completion of a secondary curriculum

(d) Original transcript of records

(e) Personal history statement

(f) Affidavit of support

(g) Alien certificate of registration (ACR)

(h) Student visa

(i) Certificate of Proficiency in English issued by the CLSU Department of English and Humanities for a fee, for students who come from countries where English is not the medium of instruction

(j) Security clearance from his/her embassy

c. Must pay a non-refundable application fee

d. Must qualify in the physical or health examination conducted by the University physician

e. Must present an approved application for admission

f. Others as prescribed by the concerned College

2. Applicants must meet all the prescribed requirements by the Department of Foreign Affairs and the BID.

3. A foreign student may be admitted based on availability of slot in the course applied for.

4. He or she must pledge to abide by and comply with the rules and regulations of the University/College.

GRADUATE PROGRAM

A DVM degree or its equivalent from a recognized institution is a requirement along with the submission of the following:

1. Duly accomplished application form

2. Original or authenticated transcript of records showing a grade point average (GPA) of at least 2.0 or its equivalent.

3. Applicants with GPA below 2.0 may be admitted on a probationary status if recommended by the department chair and approved by the dean after thorough review of the applicant's qualification to do graduate work.

4. Two letters of recommendation from former professors in the undergraduate course.

Is a Bachelor's Degree Required? no

Is this an International School? yes

ESTIMATED TUITION

Estimated Tuition Resident: Php 7,000.00 per semester

Estimated Tuition Non-Resident (International): Php 12,000.00 per semester

AVAILABLE SEATS

Resident: N/A

Non-Resident (International): n/a

VMCAS Participation: non-VMCAS

Accepts International Students? yes

Application Deadline: Last week of April every year.

UNIVERSITY OF COPENHAGEN

Email: hhd@sund.ku.dk
Website: www.sund.ku.dk

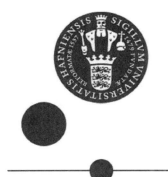

UNIVERSITY OF
COPENHAGEN

SCHOOL DESCRIPTION

The Veterinary School in Copenhagen was founded in 1773 as one of the first schools in the world. In 1856 the veterinary school was moved to its present location and at that time acquired the status of an institution of higher learning incorporating agriculture and animal science. In 2007 the Royal Veterinary and Agricultural University merged with the University of Copenhagen and was transformed into the Faculty of Life Sciences incorporating the veterinary school. The University of Copenhagen was inaugurated on 1 June 1479, after King Christian I was granted approval for its establishment by Pope Sixtus IV. Based on a German model, the university consisted of four faculties: Theology, Law, Medicine and Philosophy. Today with more than 38,000 students and more than 9,000 employees, the University of Copenhagen is the largest institution of research and education in Denmark. The purpose of the University – to quote the University Statute – is to 'conduct research and provide further education to the highest academic level'.

> The University of Copenhagen is the largest institution of research and education in Denmark.

Approximately one hundred different institutes, departments, laboratories, centers, museums, etc., form the nucleus of the University, where professors, lecturers and other academic staff, as well as most of the technical and administrative personnel, carry out their daily work, and where teaching takes place. With the opening of the totally rebuilt and modernized Small Animal University Hospital at the Frederiksberg Campus in early 2011 the Copenhagen Veterinary School including the newly built Large Animal University Hospital at the Taastrup Campus functions as one of the most modern veterinary schools with state of the art equipment.

In 2012 the Copenhagen School of Veterinary Medicine together with the School of Pharmaceutical Sciences merged with the Faculty of Health to form a new, scientifically and financially strong Faculty of Health and Medicine within the University of Copenhagen.

ORGANIZATION AND STAFF

The veterinary school encompasses 2 departments with specialized facilities, a Faculty Office and a number of general services (e.g., learning environment with audio-visual units, library, experimental farms, student facilities including several computer rooms, etc). The veterinary school has an academic staff of 276 academic staff, including 29 full professors and an administrative and support staff of 356 support staff. Most staff members communicate well in English and all academic staff members have experience in teaching veterinary medicine in English. In early 2012 all academic staff members have completed officially approved proficiency tests in English.

UNDERGRADUATE VETERINARY EDUCATION

Admission of students to the 5½-year undergraduate veterinary training program is limited to 180 each year, resulting in a total of 1100 students. They pass full examinations at the completion of each course.

RESEARCH AND POSTGRADUATE EDUCATION

Research at the School of Veterinary Medicine is the responsibility of the Vice Dean for Research and the department heads. Research which is conducted as part of the PhD programs is included in this portfolio.

QUALITY OF EDUCATION

The School of Veterinary Medicine, Faculty of Health and Medicine within the University of Copenhagen has been regularly evaluated and accredited by the European Association of Establishments of Veterinary Education since 1988 (latest accreditation in 2010).

INFORMATION ABOUT THE ADMISSION TO THE FACULTY OF VETERINARY MEDICINE FOR FOREIGN STUDENTS

In general foreign students have access to the Danish universities.

Special rules apply for the study of Veterinary Medicine. The Danish Ministry of Science has declared a numerous clauses to the DVM program. This entails that only a limited amount of students is admitted each year. The number of admission requests largely exceeds the number of allocations. Restrictions affect both Danish and foreign students. The available places are assigned by selection through interviews (50%) or based upon grades obtained in high school (50%). Letters of recommendation are neither required nor accepted.

APPLICATION TO THE DANISH DVM PROGRAM

Each year the minister of education and science lays down the number of students to be admitted to the DVM program. Currently 180 students are accepted in each class. There are two routes of application. The first is solely based upon high school grades (Quota I) and the second is based upon a mixture of high school grades, working experience and an interview (Quota II). No standardized tests are required before application. Application deadline for Quota I is 5 July 2015, and for Quota II the application deadline is 15 March 2017.

International students are referred to http://vetschool.ku.dk/english for further information about application for the Danish DVM program.

TUITION FEES AND SCHOLARSHIPS

Generally students from within the European Union do not pay tuition fee. For foreign students please refer to web site of the Ministry of Science, Technology and Innovation http://en.vtu.dk or to http://vetschool.ku.dk/english. Generally financial aid is not offered to foreign students.

RESIDENCE PERMIT

Foreign students who want to receive an academic education in Denmark need a residence permit. More information can be obtained at the Danish embassy in the country of origin.

Additionally applicants must demonstrate access to sufficient financial means. The amount varies and more detailed information should be sought at a Danish embassy.

PRE-VET PROFILE: VICTORIA TAYLOR

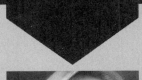

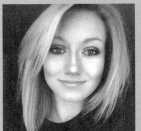

Current School Name
Western Kentucky University

What type of veterinary medicine are you interested in pursuing, and why?
I am interested in pursuing and practicing veterinary medicine predominantly with regard to companion animals. I have a passion for helping treat and prevent diseases and injuries in these animals and providing comfort and assistance to their owners. I also feel the need to help prevent further homelessness of these animals by spaying and neutering strays and attempting to find homes for those that are suitable for adoption.

What is/was your major during undergraduate school?
I am currently working toward a major in agriculture with concentrations in animal science and pre-veterinary medicine and with a chemistry minor.

What are your short-term and long-term goals?
My upcoming goals for myself are to continue upholding a 4.0 GPA at Western Kentucky University while completing my coursework, to graduate from the Honors College at Western Kentucky University, and to be accepted into Auburn University's veterinary program. My long-term goal, once I obtain my DVM, is to establish my own private practice dealing with companion animals. As part of having my own clinic, I also would like to establish an animal shelter that can help provide care to strays and homeless animals that really need it and to help those animals find suitable forever homes.

What are you doing as an applicant/pre-vet to prepare for veterinary school?
In order to prepare for veterinary school, I am enrolled in the pre-veterinary curriculum at Western Kentucky University. I currently volunteer at the local Humane Society Shelter once a week to gain experience working with the animals as well as helping socialize them so they are more likely to be adopted. In addition, I am seeking a position to job shadow a practicing veterinarian so that I may gain experience and a better understanding of the daily activities of the career and what it takes.

What extracurricular activities are you involved in currently?
I am a member of both the Pre-Vet Club and the Block and Bridle Club at Western Kentucky University.

How old were you when you first became interested in being a veterinarian?
When I was a little girl, I always played doctor to my stuffed animals, and so I think I was interested in being a veterinarian from a very early age. That interest really came to light when I was 12 years old. My dog had to be euthanized due to cancer that had spread throughout her body, and that experience really made me consider a career as a veterinarian because I saw firsthand the help and care that I could possibly provide. It was a difficult experience but I understood the situation, and from then on, it was my dream to become a veterinarian.

Please describe your various experiences in preparation for applying to veterinary school.
Once a week, I volunteer at the local animal shelter by socializing with the animals—specifically playing with the cats and walking dogs. It is really a rewarding experience because not only am I helping these animals by socializing them so that they may be more readily adopted, but they also help me by giving me experience. In my animal science course, I have gained experience in vaccinating cattle and giving dewormer to horses. I also have been able to learn from and witness the processes involved in castration and necropsy. In addition, I have researched various schools and requirements in order to best prepare myself for applying.

What characteristics are you looking for in a veterinary school?
When looking into veterinary schools, it is really important to me to best prepare myself for the future, and so I look heavily into the curriculum and success rates on the NAVLE. In addition, I look at financial aid and scholarship opportunities, especially for a Kentucky resident.

What advice do you have for other pre-veterinary students?
It is important to gain as much experience as possible in order to familiarize yourself with the career and establish relationships with other veterinarians.

SEOUL NATIONAL UNIVERSITY

Email Address: snuadmit@snu.ac.kr
Website: http://en.snu.ac.kr/apply/info

서 울 대 학 교
SEOUL NATIONAL UNIVERSITY

SCHOOL DESCRIPTION

Seoul National University honors the ideals of liberal education and aims to teach students a lifelong love of learning that will form the basis for continuous personal growth.

At the same time it is committed to preparing students to work and live in an increasingly competitive global environment. As South Korea's first national university, Seoul National University has a tradition of standing up for democracy and peace on the Korean peninsula.

Graduates have long served as public servants in key positions of the Korean government. In teaching, research, and public service, Seoul National University continues to set the standard of excellence.

The mission of Seoul National University in the twenty-first century is to create a vibrant intellectual community where students and scholars join together in building the future. As Korea's leading research university, Seoul National University is committed to diversifying its student body and faculty, fostering global exchange, and promoting path-breaking research in all fields of knowledge.

In teaching, research, and public service, Seoul National University continues to set the standard of excellence.

2016 FALL ADMISSIONS TIMELINE

The dates and deadlines below are for the application to the program that starts in Fall 2016

ONLINE APPLICATION

Period : January 11 (Mon)~February 18 (Thu), 2016
   *Note that the entrance to the program is in Sep, 2016.

SUBMISSION OF DOCUMENTS

Period: January 11 (Mon)~February 29 (Fri), 2016
   *After completing the online application, the required documents should arrive at the SNU Office of Admissions by due date.

PERFORMANCE TEST

International admission type II (Undergraduate) applicant who received the entire education abroad applying for the following programs: Fine Arts, Music, or Physical Education, may be subject to a performance test.

   *In such a case, the corresponding College/Department will individually notify the applicants for futher details.

ANNOUNCEMENT OF ADMISSIONS DECISION

April 27 (Wed), 2016
   *Results will be posted on the SNU website NOTICE

REGISTRATION

August 2016 (TBA)
   *Either at the branches of NongHyup Bank, Shinhan Bank, Woori Bank nationwide or via virtual account transfer

KOREAN PROFICIENCY TEST AMONG THE ADMITTED STUDENTS

August 2016 (TBA)
   SNU website will indicate those who are required to take the Korean proficiency Test on the admission result announcement screen.

• For further information about application process and admissions, please make an inquiry to Office of admissions' email address. (snuadmit@snu.ac.kr) or (http://en.snu.ac.kr/apply/info)

ST. MATTHEW'S UNIVERSITY

Email Address: admissions@stmatthews.edu
Website: www.stmatthews.edu

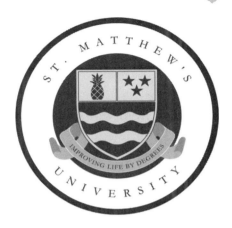

SCHOOL DESCRIPTION

St. Matthew's University School of Veterinary Medicine is located on beautiful Grand Cayman in the Caribbean. Grand Cayman is the fifth largest financial district in the world and has a highly developed infrastructure which is very comparable to the United States. It is also one of the safest islands in the Caribbean, boasting one of the lowest crime and poverty rates. Grand Cayman has hundreds of restaurants, scores of banks, world-class hotels, and many opportunities for boating, diving, horseback riding, and other recreation. The island is less than an hours flight from Miami, and also has direct flights from Atlanta, Chicago, Charlotte, Houston, Tampa, Toronto, Washington D.C., and other locations.

> Throughout your ten semesters at St. Matthew's University, we will support all aspects of your education and life.

At SMU, we are as committed to your dreams as you are. Throughout your ten semesters with us, we will do everything we can to ensure your success by supporting all aspects of your education and life, including:

Focus on Teaching: Dedicated, talented faculty whose time commitments are focused on teaching and mentoring.

Student Mentors: Student mentors understand about adjusting to life in veterinary school, and are eager to see you succeed.

Very Low Student to Faculty Ratio: With a student to faculty ratio of less than five to one, you will have an unprecedented level of faculty support and attention.

We limit each incoming cohort of students to a maximum of 25.

Best Value: Most affordable tuition of any Caribbean veterinary school.

Accelerated Schedule: Complete your pre-clinical education on Grand Cayman in just 28 months, and then return to the U.S. or Canada for clinical training, with the ability to complete vet school in just over three years.

SMU's modern, state-of-the-art main campus is located across the street from beautiful Seven Mile Beach, and boasts wireless technology throughout the bright, air-conditioned classrooms, labs, library, and student lounges. SMU also has a Clinical Teaching Facility which hosts surgery, medicine and clinical skills training as well as anatomy and pathology laboratories. Students have the opportunity to travel to local farms with veterinary staff from the Cayman Department of Agriculture. Our students spend seven (7) semesters on Grand Cayman and their final months in clinical programs at one of our many AVMA-accredited Clinical Program Affiliate Schools in the United States and Canada.

There arc significant opportunities for students to gain experience with exotic species through our collaborations with the Cayman Turtle Farm, Central Caribbean Marine Institute, Dolphin Discovery, the Blue Iguana Project and the Marine Research Program.

APPLICATION INFORMATION

We welcome applications from any qualified candidate who dreams of become a veterinarian. For specific application information (availability, deadlines, fees, transferring to SMU and VMCAS participation), please refer to the contact information above.

SUMMARY OF ADMISSIONS PROCEDURES

Timetable

Application deadlines: None. Rolling admissions. Three incoming cohorts per year.

Interviews: Held in person or via telephone/videoconference.

School begins: August, January, May (three start dates per year).

Deposit (to hold a place in class): $500.00

Deferments: Considered on an individual basis.

Transfer applications for admission with advanced standings are welcome. Transfer credits (advance standing) may be awarded at the discretion of the University. No transfers are permitted alter than beginning of Semester 5.

Seats generally available: Maximum of 30 (total) seats available per incoming cohort to ensure exceptional level of faculty support for students.

ENTRANCE REQUIREMENTS

All prerequisite courses must be completed prior to matriculation.

Is a Bachelor's Degree Required? no

Is this an International School? yes

ESTIMATED TUITION

Estimated Tuition Resident: Pre-Clinical Sciences (Grand Cayman): $14,125

Estimated Tuition Contract: Clinical Sciences (Clinical Affiliates): $21,750

Estimated Tuition Non-Resident: Additional Fees: $0

AVAILABLE SEATS

Resident: 0

Contract: 0

Non-Resident: 25, 3 times per year

TEST REQUIREMENTS

Graduate Record Examination (GRE), general test, is not required but is recommended.

VMCAS Participation: non-VMCAS

Accepts International Students? yes

ADDITIONAL INFORMATION

The admissions team at SMU wants to get to know you! To us, you are much more than a GPA or GRE score. We want to know about you as a person because ultimately, that is what will determine the kind of veterinarian you will be. We want to support you in your dram of becoming a veterinarian, and we welcome your application!

Application Deadline: rolling

UNIVERSITY OF TOKYO*

Graduate School of Agricultural and Life Sciences
The University of Tokyo
1-1-1, Yayoi, Bunkyo-ku, Tokyo, 113-8657

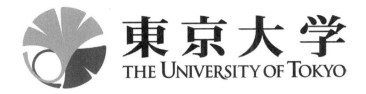

TOKYO

SCHOOL DESCRIPTION

Veterinary medicine covers wide areas of life sciences, not only medicine for animals but also biology of mammals and higher vertebrates. In the Department of Veterinary Medicine, most advanced research is being carried out at molecular, cellular and in vivo levels, in order to fully understand vital processes of normal and diseased animals. Veterinary medicine has two aspects of science: basic science to understand the mechanisms underlying biological phenomena, and applied science to satisfy the social demands for maintenance and improvement of human welfare and productivity of domestic animals. This department collaborates with the veterinary medical center located on the Yayoi campus. This center is facilitated with the latest and most advanced medical instruments, and plays an important role as an advanced veterinary hospital in this area.

> The Department of Veterinary Medicine collaborates with the veterinary medical center located on the Yayoi campus.

FOR MORE INFORMATION

For more information about the University of Tokyo's Veterinary Medicine Program, please go to the following website: http://www.u-tokyo.ac.jp/en/admissions-and-programs/graduate-and-research/graduate-schools/agricultural.html

---

東京大学
THE UNIVERSITY OF TOKYO

POLICIES ON ADVANCED STANDING

Transfers are permitted to most colleges of veterinary medicine in the United States under specified conditions. Typical requirements include a vacancy in the class, completion of all prerequisite requirements, and compatible curricula. Following is a listing of schools and some of the conditions under which they will consider a transfer from another veterinary college with advanced standing. More detailed information may be obtained by writing to the individual schools in which you have an interest.

UNITED STATES

UNIVERSITY OF CALIFORNIA, DAVIS

Applications may be considered if available positions exist within the third-year classes. Currently, each class in the DVM program of the School of Veterinary Medicine shall consist of no more than 138 students.

1. The applicant must have a strong academic record in his/her undergraduate program.
2. The applicant must be currently enrolled in an AVMA-accredited DVM program and must be in excellent academic and ethical standing in that program. The specific minimum benchmark will be that the applicant is in the top quartile of students in the Veterinary School in which the applicant is currently enrolled as determined by GPA or class rank.
3. The applicant must have completed veterinary course work equivalent to that expected of the students in the DVM program of the School of Veterinary Medicine, UC Davis, who will be in the same academic class.
4. The applicant has a valid reason for requesting admission in advanced standing.

UNIVERSITY OF FLORIDA

1. An opening must exist in the second- or third-year class.
2. Students are only rarely considered for advanced standing based on exceptional personal circumstances.
3. Student must be enrolled in an AVMA accredited college.
4. Student must meet all prerequisites for admission as a first-year student (including GRE® scores).
5. The curricula of the two schools must be sufficiently alike to allow a student to enter without deficiencies in academic background.

6. Applicants must have a letter approving transfer from their dean or associate dean.

UNIVERSITY OF GEORGIA

1. Priority is given to Georgia residents, followed by contract state residents, then all other applicants.
2. Applicants will be considered for entry into the DVM degree program up to the third year of the curriculum, when and if space is available, as defined by the Admissions Committee.
3. Applications must include official transcripts of all completed veterinary and pre-veterinary coursework and a letter of support written by a senior administrator of the school in which the applicant is currently enrolled stating the applicant is currently in good academic standing.
4. No individual is eligible for transfer who has been dismissed or is on probation at any other school or college for deficiency in scholarship or because of misconduct.

UNIVERSITY OF ILLINOIS

1. Transfer students will only be considered for the beginning of the second year of veterinary medicine and only if transfer seats become available in that class.
2. All prerequisite science courses must be completed prior to the request for transfer.
3. Minimum grade requirements include:
   cumulative and science GPAs of 2.75 on a 4.00 scale (doesn't include veterinary work); results of the Graduate Record Examination General Test completed within the last two years.
4. Student must complete the same preveterinary coursework as required for students accepted to the first year of the program.
5. Student must be in good academic standing.
6. To be considered for transfer, a student must present credentials for preprofessional work that fulfill the University of Illinois College of Veterinary Medicine requirements for first-year entry.
7. Complete information and an application can be found at www.vetmed.illinois.edu/asa/brochure.

COLORADO STATE UNIVERSITY

Transfer is dependent on position openings in the year into which the student transfers (most transfers will involve the loss of a year because of differences in school curricula). Candidate must:

1. have successfully completed at least the first year (equivalent of two semesters) of veterinary curriculum at an AVMA accredited college of veterinary medicine.

AND

2. have obtained the equivalent of a 3.0 cumulative GPA in your veterinary program AND must not have received a D, F, or unsatisfactory grade of any kind since enrolling in veterinary school.

AND

3. have a preveterinary academic record comparable to currently enrolled DVM students.

AND

4. provide evidence of noncognitive attributes comparable to currently enrolled DVM students.

If a veterinary student with an interest in transferring to CSU's DVM program meets ALL of the above minimum requirements, he/she may apply to the DVM program. To apply for transfer to CSU's Veterinary Program, please see http://csu-cvmbs.colostate.edu /Documents/dvm-policy-transfer-students.pdf.

CORNELL UNIVERSITY

1. Students are considered for advanced standing in rare and exceptional circumstances. Each request for transfer is considered on an individual basis.
2. Transfer students will be considered if an opening exists in the second-year class. Students seeking advanced standing may enter the DVM program at two points: at the beginning of the second year of study, or mid-way through the second year, at the beginning of the fourth (Spring) semester of study.
3. Students seeking advanced standing must be enrolled in an AVMA-accredited veterinary college.
4. The curricula of the two schools must be sufficiently similar to allow students to enter without deficiencies in their academic background.
5. Students must meet all pre-veterinary requirements for first-year entry at the College of Veterinary Medicine at Cornell University (including GRE scores, prerequisite coursework, animal and veterinary experience), and may not have any failing grades on their veterinary transcript.
6. Scores from the Graduate Record Examination (GRE) or Medical College Admissions Test (MCAT) may not be older than five years.
7. Applicants seeking advanced standing must include a letter from their Associate Dean certifying that the student is in good academic standing, has not been on academic probation, and has not been subject to any disciplinary action or dismissal for any reason.

8. Applicants are required to have completed at least two full semesters at the institution from which the transfer is requested. Only veterinary coursework completed at an AVMA-accredited institution will be considered.
9. After analyzing the academic background of the applicant, the Admissions Committee will place each accepted transfer student in the semester of study in the DVM curriculum deemed most appropriate. (Veterinary course syllabi will be required at time of application).

IOWA STATE UNIVERSITY

Acceptance of students for advanced standing is on the recommendation of the Academic Standards Committee. Space must be available in the class to which the student is applying. See website, http://vetmed.iastate .edu/student/future-dvm-students/apply-to-the-college /transfer-admissions/application-process.

KANSAS STATE UNIVERSITY

Acceptance of students for transfer is on recommendation of the Admissions Committee on a space-available basis.

LOUISIANA STATE UNIVERSITY

1. There must be a vacancy in the class.
2. The curricula must be compatible.
3. The student must be in good academic standing with at least a 3.2 GPA in veterinary coursework at his/her present college.
4. Admission is limited to the second year of the program and only into the fall semester.
5. Each request for transfer is considered on a case-by-case basis.
6. To initiate the transfer process, please carefully read the DVM Transfer Guidelines information at http://www.lsu.edu/vetmed/dvm_admissions/how _to_apply/transfers.php.

MICHIGAN STATE UNIVERSITY

1. Admission consideration is offered only to those current matriculants in professional veterinary curricula who believe that there are extenuating circumstances that would precipitate significant undue hardship if they continue at their current institution.
2. Applicants requesting a transfer must contact the Dean of Academic and Student Affairs at the school they are currently attending and notify him or her of their intent.

3. Applicants must also demonstrate quality academic performance throughout their professional school enrollment.
4. The curricula of the two schools must be sufficiently alike to allow a student to enter the second-year class without deficiencies in academic background.
5. All selection criteria for regular applicants apply to transfer applicants.
6. Priority is given to Michigan residents.
7. Applicants who have previously been denied admission to MSU CVM will not be considered for transfer admissions.
8. Space must be available.
9. AVMA accreditation of current school is considered.

UNIVERSITY OF MINNESOTA

1. Transfer students are accepted on a space available basis. The Admissions Committee will place each applicant in the year or semester of the curriculum deemed appropriate after analysis of equivalency of the required courses involved.
2. No academic work or standing will be accepted from DVM curricula other than those deemed accredited by the American Veterinary Medical Association.
3. All applicants must be U.S. citizens or holders of appropriate visas.
4. All applicants are required to have finished at least one full academic year at the institution from which transfer is requested and must be in good academic standing at the time of discontinuance according to written verification from the institution.
5. All applicants must have achieved a cumulative GPA of 3.00 (of 4.00) for the required courses at the initial institution.
6. Please visit the following website for more details: http://www.cvm.umn.edu/students/prospective -dvm-students/how-to-apply/Transfer-Student -Information/index.htm.

MISSISSIPPI STATE UNIVERSITY

The Mississippi State University College of Veterinary Medicine accepts, on a limited basis, transfer students from other veterinary medical colleges to fill vacancies in the freshmen or sophomore classes. Transfer guidelines are as follows:

From a veterinary school not accredited by the AVMA:

Applicants for transfer into the second semester of the first year must have completed coursework equivalent to coursework taught in the first semester of the first year at MSU-CVM.

Applicants for transfer into the first semester of the second year must have   completed coursework equivalent to coursework taught in the first year at MSU-CVM.

Applicants for transfer into the second semester of the second year must have completed coursework equivalent to all coursework taught in the first three semesters at MSU-CVM plus have had equivalent surgery laboratories.

From a veterinary school accredited by the AVMA:

Applicants are considered on a case-by-case basis with regard to length of time in current program.

General:

Any applicant considered for transfer admission must be in good academic standing (defined as being eligible to continue at current school from current point in the curriculum), never have failed a course while in veterinary medical school, never have been dismissed from a veterinary school and must have completed at least a full academic year at current veterinary school

Any applicants considered for transfer admission will be required to attend an interview at Mississippi State University.

Typically, transfer applicants are not accepted into our program at a point later than first semester of the sophomore year. Accordingly, if a student should pursue application to Mississippi State University College of Veterinary Medicine and be accepted, it would be necessary for that student to complete at least two years at Mississippi State University to be eligible for a degree.

Students accepted for transfer are required to meet the current computer requirements of the college.

For more information, contact Tonya Calmes, Admissions Assistant, 662-325-4161, tcalmes@cvm.msstate.edu.

UNIVERSITY OF MISSOURI

1. Must be a vacancy in the class.
2. Will consider students who are U.S. citizens or holders of permanent alien visas and who have finished at least two years in a college of veterinary medicine that is AVMA accredited.
3. Students must be in good academic standing, never been denied admission from the University of Missouri for a first year position, and submit a letter of reference from the dean's office of the present college is required.

NORTH CAROLINA STATE UNIVERSITY

1. Must be a vacancy in the class.
2. Consideration by the Admission Committee on an individual basis.
3. Curricula must be compatible.
4. A letter from the dean of the current school certifying the applicant's academic standing.
5. Letter of recommendation from a faculty member at the original college.
6. Only accept transfers from AVMA accredited colleges.
7. At least 50% of DVM credit hours must be completed at North Carolina State in order to earn a North Carolina State University degree.

THE OHIO STATE UNIVERSITY

The Ohio State University does not accept transfer students.

OKLAHOMA STATE UNIVERSITY

Transfer students are considered. Each application is evaluated on an individual basis. See website for transfer guide: http://www.cvhs.okstate.edu

OREGON STATE UNIVERSITY

Admission of students with advanced standing is considered only in certain circumstances, and each case is considered on an individual basis.

UNIVERSITY OF PENNSYLVANIA

PennVet does not consider transfer applications.

PURDUE UNIVERSITY

1. Positions must be available in the relevant class.
2. Student must be in good academic standing in his/her present program.
3. Students must have completed 1–2 years of DVM courses with an **exceptional** academic record in those courses.
4. Veterinary medical curricula must be compatible.
5. Student must have support of the administration from the program in which he/she is currently enrolled.

Please visit the following website for more specific detail: http://www.vet.purdue.edu/dvm/files/documents/transfer_policy.pdf

UNIVERSITY OF TENNESSEE

Admission of students with advanced standing (transfer) may be considered for unique circumstances on a case-by-case basis.

1. Position(s) must be available in the class into which one would like to matriculate.

2. Curricula of the two schools must be sufficiently alike to allow a student to matriculate without deficiencies in his/her academic background.
3. The applicant's academic dean must provide a letter approving transfer and indicating that the student is in good standing at his/her current college/school of veterinary medicine.
4. Admission is usually limited to the second semester of the first year of the DVM curriculum except for exceptional circumstances.
5. Letters of reference are required.

The Admissions Committee will review applicant credentials and interview those determined to best meet admission criteria.

TEXAS A&M UNIVERSITY

Students requesting advanced standing must meet the following requirements:

1. Must have completed all previous professional veterinary courses in an AVMA accredited college of veterinary medicine.
2. Must have successfully completed the academic term preceding the semester into which student requests admission.
3. Must comply with all requirements for transfer into the university as described in the current catalog.
4. May request transfer only into the second through seventh semesters of the professional curriculum.
5. At the time of matriculation the student must certify by letter that he/she has not been convicted of crimes in the period from first enrollment in the college of veterinary medicine from which the student desires transfer until date of matriculation at Texas A&M University.
6. To request transfer consideration, the student must meet all requirements as posted on the College website at http://vetmed.tamu.edu/dvm/future/transferring.

TUFTS UNIVERSITY

Applicants from other veterinary schools are considered. Students with advanced standing are admitted if and when space becomes available in the second-year class. The application deadline is June 1 for the following September. Please refer to our web site for details: http://www.tufts.edu/vet

TUSKEGEE UNIVERSITY

General: In most instances, transfer of a DVM student from their current program into the DVM program at Tuskegee will not be possible. However, in some cases transfer can be accomplished if a series of criteria can be met.

Criteria required for transfer: There are six specific criteria that must be met in order for a DVM student matriculating at another veterinary school or college of veterinary medicine to transfer into the DVM program at Tuskegee University College of Veterinary Medicine (TUCVM). These criteria are listed below.

1. The student seeking transfer to TUCVM must be currently enrolled in a school or college of veterinary medicine that is fully accredited by the American Veterinary Medical Association Counsel ob Education,

2. The student seeking to transfer to TUCVM must be in good academic standing at the veterinary school or college they are matriculating.

3. The DVM curriculum at the perspective transferees' school or college of matriculation must be sufficiently similar to the DVM curriculum at TUCVM to make transfer possible.

4. The perspective transferees' reason(s) for wanting to effect a transfer from their current DVM program to the DVM program at TUCVM must be evaluated and deemed an appropriate reason(s).

5. The perspective transferee must have either the Associate Dean For Academic Affairs or the Dean of their current DVM program submit a letter to the Director of Veterinary Admissions at TUCVM which specifically reaffirms the reason(s) for wanting to transfer and which also states that the perspective transferee is not under any present non-academic probationary status or under any present or pending disciplinary action(s).

6. The transfer must be approved by the Dean of the Tuskegee University College of Veterinary Medicine, Nursing, and Allied Health.

VIRGINIA-MARYLAND
COLLEGE OF VETERINARY MEDICINE

VMRCVM accepts students for advanced standing on the recommendation of the Admissions Committee on a space-available basis.

WASHINGTON STATE UNIVERSITY

Admission of students with advanced standing is considered only in very specific and unique circumstances, and each case is considered on an individual basis.

UNIVERSITY OF WISCONSIN

Wisconsin does not accept advanced standing students for admission.

INTERNATIONAL

ATLANTIC VETERINARY COLLEGE AT THE UNIVERSITY OF PRINCE EDWARD ISLAND

Applicants who have completed all or portions of a veterinary medical program may apply for advanced standing to the second year of the DVM program.

Applicants for advanced standing must present evidence of educational accomplishments and may be required to address missing courses or competencies expected of our incoming second-year students. Students admitted with advanced standing must begin the college year in September.

The candidate must file a formal application and may be interviewed by the Admissions Committee and possibly other faculty. Places for admission to the college with advanced standing are limited and depend on vacancies.

It is imperative that the Admissions Committee have detailed and translated summaries of veterinary medical academic programs and accomplishments for those seeking advanced placement from schools in foreign countries.

Advanced-standing applications should be on file and completed as early as possible and no later than January 1. Candidates are strongly encouraged to visit the website http://stage.upei.ca/avcpolicies/files/avcpolicies/avcaa_adm0004.pdf.

MASSEY UNIVERSITY

Applications for admission with advanced standing will only be considered by students enrolled in a veterinary program with a compatible curriculum, and pending an available space in the appropriate stage of the program. Applicants should contact vetschool@massey.ac.nz to apply for advanced standing.

MURDOCH UNIVERSITY

Applications for advanced standing will only be considered from students whose studies have been completed in a DVM program. Applicants are required to apply formally for advanced standing and provide the necessary documentation to allow for a full comparison between the previous study and Murdoch University's unit requirements. Prior courses must duplicate or substantially overlap multiple factors including breadth and depth of content, duration, objectives, assessment, context, and academic standard (level of intellectual effort required) for exemption to be granted.

ST. MATTHEW'S UNIVERSITY

Applications for admission with advanced standing are welcomed from students from veterinary schools recognized by the American Veterinary Medical Association (AVMA) and/or the American Association of Veterinary State Boards (AAVSB). Transfer applicants must submit a complete application package to ensure a timely review. Acceptance of transfer credit is at the discretion of St. Matthew's University.

UNIVERSITY OF CALGARY

Applications for admission to advanced semesters may be considered from students who have been enrolled in DVM programs at other institutions, subject to the availability of spaces in the DVM Program and the academic standing of the candidate. When places are available, candidates may be asked to present themselves for an interview and may be asked to pass examinations on subject matter in the veterinary curriculum. Applicants are advised that vacancies are rare and that restrictions on residency and citizenship status may be applied.

THE UNIVERSITY OF QUEENSLAND

Applications for advanced standing will only be considered from students whose studies have been completed in a veterinary program with a compatible curriculum, and where a space is available in the appropriate stage of the program. Please refer to the University of Queensland Policy 3.50.03 - Credit for Previous Studies and Recognised Prior Learning (http://ppl.app.uq.edu.au) or contact the School directly (vetenquiries@uq.edu.au).

UNIVERSITY OF SASKATCHEWAN

Applications for admission with advanced standing will only be considered if a vacancy in the Year II class develops. Students applying for advanced standing must meet the normal residency requirements and must be enrolled in a program that has a compatible curriculum. Applicants are required to complete a formal application form and, dependent on their academic record, will be considered for an interview. Part of the interview will be an assessment of their current knowledge. If English is not their first language, applicants will also be required to submit a TOEFL score. Admission is not considered beyond the second year of the program.

Enrolled First-Year Students
by Resident vs. Non-Resident Status

AAVMC Internal Reports
2016-2017

■ Resident Students ■ Residents attending Private In-State CVMs ■ Non-Resident Students

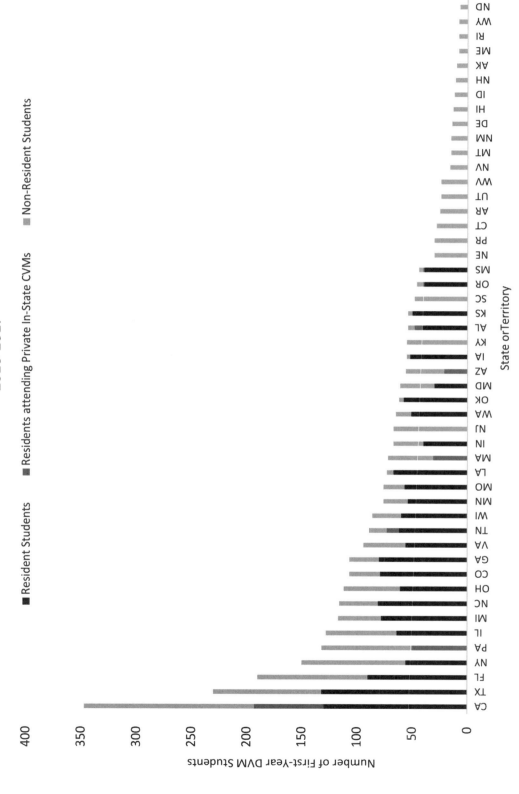

Total class size = 3,372

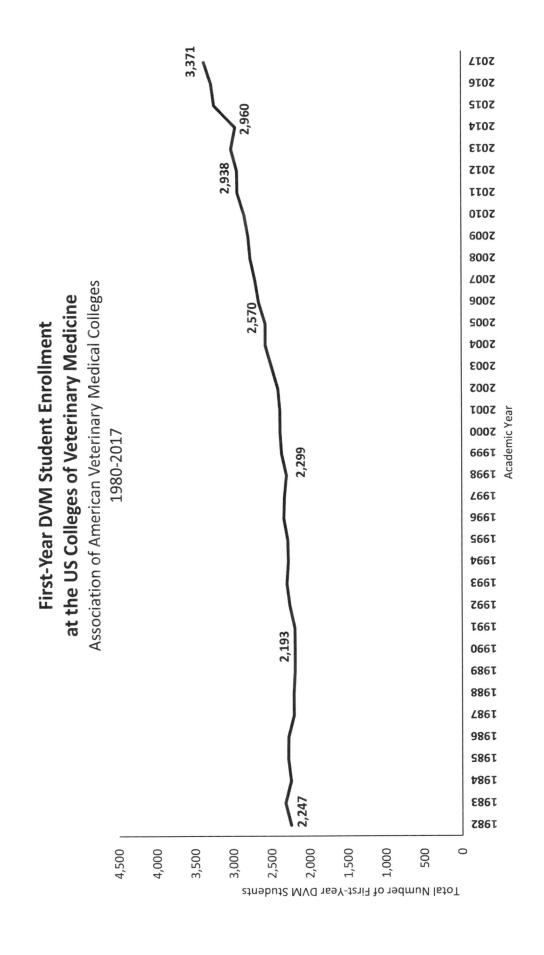

First-Year DVM Student Enrollment
at the US Colleges of Veterinary Medicine
Association of American Veterinary Medical Colleges
1980-2017

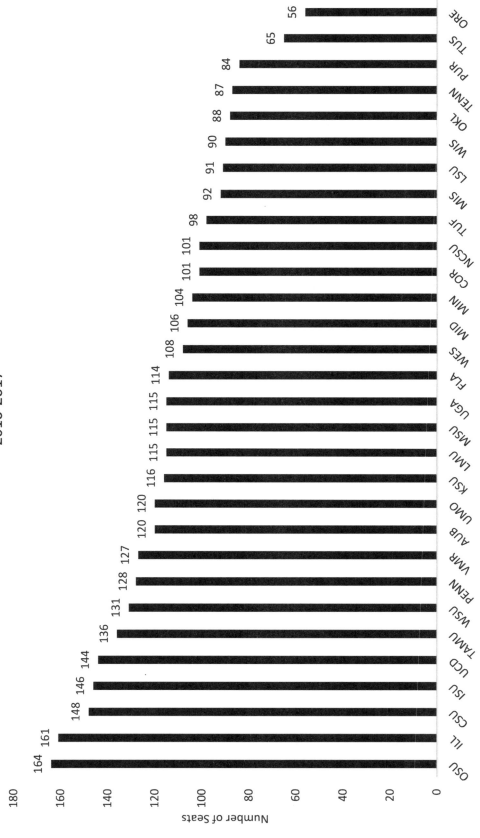

Number of Seats in the First-Year Class

By US College of Veterinary Medicine
AAVMC Internal Reports
2016-2017

Number of Seats

OSU 164
ILL 161
CSU 148
ISU 146
UCD 144
TAMU 136
WSU 131
PENN 128
VMR 127
AUB 120
UMO 120
KSU 116
LMU 115
MSU 115
UGA 115
FLA 114
WES 108
MID 106
MIN 104
COR 101
NCSU 101
TUF 98
MIS 92
LSU 91
WIS 90
OKL 88
TENN 87
PUR 84
TUS 65
ORE 56

US College of Veterinary Medicine

Total class size = 3,372

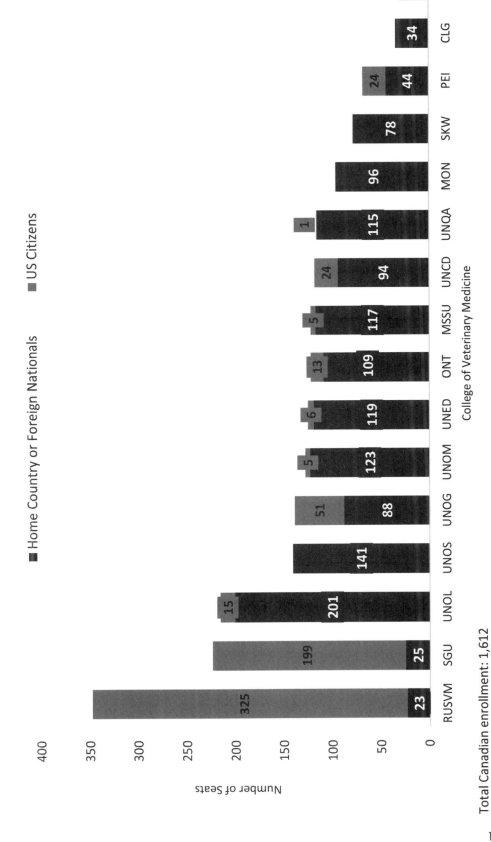

Number of Seats in the First Year Class

By Canadian & International
College of Veterinary Medicine
AAVMC Internal Reports
2016-2017

■ Home Country or Foreign Nationals ■ US Citizens

Number of Seats

College of Veterinary Medicine

College	Home Country or Foreign Nationals	US Citizens
RUSVM	325	23
SGU	199	25
UNOL	201	15
UNOS	141	
UNOG	88	51
UNOM	123	5
UNED	119	6
ONT	109	13
MSSU	117	5
UNCD	94	24
UNQA	115	1
MON	96	
SKW	78	
PEI	44	24
CLG	34	
MDU	30	

Total Canadian enrollment: 1,612
Total International enrollment: 7,826 (Lyon, UNAM & Utrecht did not report enrollment.)

185

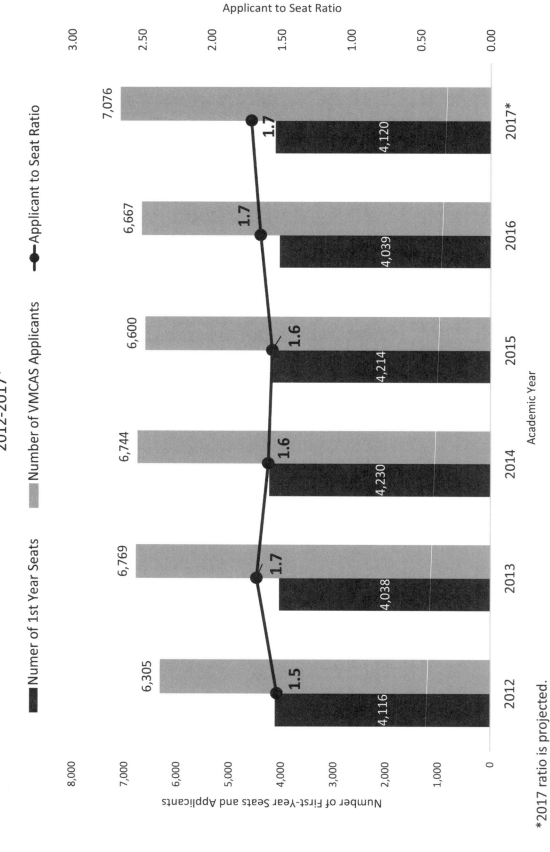

VMCAS Applicants and First-Year Seats
US and International Institutions
AAVMC Internal Reports
2012-2017*

■ Numer of 1st Year Seats   ■ Number of VMCAS Applicants   ●—Applicant to Seat Ratio

Applicant to Seat Ratio

Academic Year

Number of First-Year Seats and Applicants

*2017 ratio is projected.

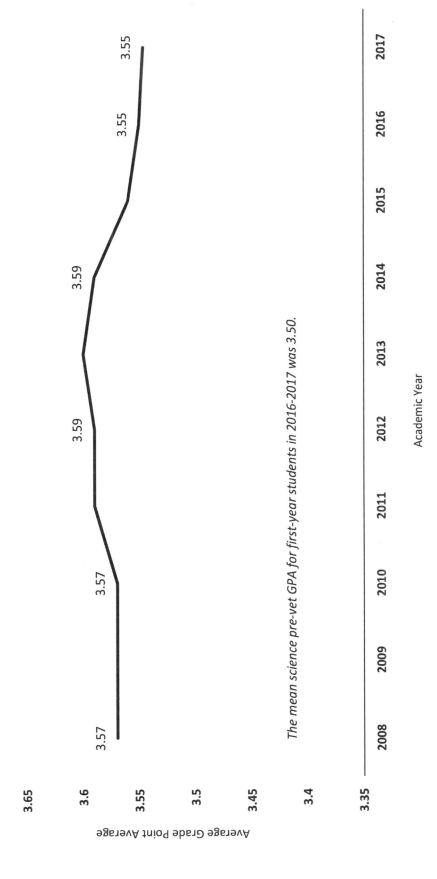

First-Year Student Pre-Vet GPA

AAVMC Internal Reports
2008-2017

3.57

3.57

3.59

3.59

3.55

3.55

The mean science pre-vet GPA for first-year students in 2016-2017 was 3.50.

Average Grade Point Average

Academic Year

GPA is calculated on a 4.0 scale.
Line chart is shown on an excerpted scale of 3.35 to 3.75.

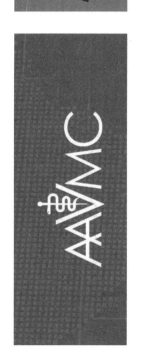

Additional Applicant Information

- **Average Years of Pre-professional Preparation**
  - 4.4 Years
- **Average Age for First-Year Enrollees**
  - 23.3 Years
- **GRE Scores – Class of 2019**
  - Average Verbal Percentile= 65.9
  - Average Quantitative Score = 56.7
  - Average Writing Score = 59.6
- **Degree status of Class of 2019 at admission**
  - No Degree Completed = 6.6%
  - BS/BA Completed = 87.7%
  - MS/MA Competed = 5.3%
  - PhD Completed = .4%
- **Percentage of Applicants Who Apply as Non-Residents**
  - 80.1%